Psychology of Wounds and Wound Care in Clinical Practice

Dominic Upton • Penney Upton

Psychology of Wounds and Wound Care in Clinical Practice

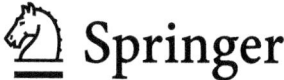

Dominic Upton
Faculty of Health
University of Canberra
Canberra
Aust Capital Terr
Australia

Penney Upton
Institute of Health and Society
University of Worcester
Worcester
UK

ISBN 978-3-319-09652-0   ISBN 978-3-319-09653-7 (eBook)
DOI 10.1007/978-3-319-09653-7
Springer Cham Heidelberg New York Dordrecht London

Library of Congress Control Number: 2014952329

© Springer International Publishing Switzerland 2015
This work is subject to copyright. All rights are reserved by the Publisher, whether the whole or part of the material is concerned, specifically the rights of translation, reprinting, reuse of illustrations, recitation, broadcasting, reproduction on microfilms or in any other physical way, and transmission or information storage and retrieval, electronic adaptation, computer software, or by similar or dissimilar methodology now known or hereafter developed. Exempted from this legal reservation are brief excerpts in connection with reviews or scholarly analysis or material supplied specifically for the purpose of being entered and executed on a computer system, for exclusive use by the purchaser of the work. Duplication of this publication or parts thereof is permitted only under the provisions of the Copyright Law of the Publisher's location, in its current version, and permission for use must always be obtained from Springer. Permissions for use may be obtained through RightsLink at the Copyright Clearance Center. Violations are liable to prosecution under the respective Copyright Law.
The use of general descriptive names, registered names, trademarks, service marks, etc. in this publication does not imply, even in the absence of a specific statement, that such names are exempt from the relevant protective laws and regulations and therefore free for general use.
While the advice and information in this book are believed to be true and accurate at the date of publication, neither the authors nor the editors nor the publisher can accept any legal responsibility for any errors or omissions that may be made. The publisher makes no warranty, express or implied, with respect to the material contained herein.

Printed on acid-free paper

Springer is part of Springer Science+Business Media (www.springer.com)

Foreword I

The Lindsay Leg Club model is based on one in which patients are empowered to take ownership of their care, alleviate their suffering and reduce the stigma attached to their condition. It also seeks to further advance education in all aspects of leg health among sufferers, carers, the general public and the healthcare professions. As president of the Lindsay Leg Club, I am therefore glad that Dominic and Penney have asked me to write this preface for their book. I know that patients with wounds and the members of our Leg Clubs across the country and beyond will be satisfied that their concerns are being listened to and their voices heard and that this is reflected here in this book.

Care of those with wounds, especially the care of chronic wounds, is an area of practice that has received much attention over recent years. In part this is due to the significant impact it can have on the costs to the health service, nursing practice and, most importantly, to the patient themselves and their family. This interest has also come about because of the increasing number of patients with such wounds and the considerable economic cost that this brings to society and the health service. As a result of increased interest the amount of research, education and training has also significantly increased. Much of this, quite rightly, has been on the medical and nursing care of those with wounds. Unfortunately, the focus on the psychological and social aspects associated with chronic wounds has been largely ignored. Although some pioneering work exploring quality of life and pain occurred in the 1990s, much of the work exploring the patient experience has been sadly neglected – until now.

Dominic has done much to promote this research and his work has looked at how people live with a wound – what issues confront individuals with chronic wounds, what their experience of treatment is, and, more recently, learning from those with wounds on how best to support others in a similar position. All of this research has one goal in mind – to improve the experience of those with chronic wounds, for which all of us are grateful. He has now decided to work with Penney to bring together their experience and expertise in this book, *Psychology of Wounds and Wound Care in Clinical Practice* – a timely and important book that will serve heath care practitioners well now and for many years to come.

He is recognised both nationally and internationally as a key leader in shaping and changing management relating to wound and leg ulcer care and is widely acknowledged as an expert in the innovative and specialised area of patient centred care. He has shown remarkable tenacity in overcoming barriers and preconceptions, leading by example through his contribution to research, practice and education.

Dominic's presentations at conferences and educational events inspire and motivate, and his ability to use humour to illustrate key points is very effective. He encourages colleagues and teams within the clinical and academic fraternity to expand and develop their knowledge and skills. So much of the Dominic's work is unique that it is difficult to highlight specific aspects, but he has developed and enhanced services with flair and originality, empowering and changing the lives of countless patients, allowing them to enjoy a better quality of life.

Penney is internationally renowned in her own right for her work on quality of life and well-being. She is now bringing this expertise to the field of chronic wounds and leg ulcer care. Her presentations at conferences and training events have highlighted her knowledge and commitment to this area. Both authors are dedicated to improving the service and thereby the lives of people with wounds.

The contents of this book are exactly what is needed and one that focuses on both the negative aspects of wounds – the pain and stress associated with the condition and its treatment, to the factors that can be beneficial and protective – social activities for example. It is important to be positive, to appreciate that with support people can (and do) live with their wounds. With appropriate medical and nursing care, wounds can be successfully treated and managed. Importantly, with psychological support people can value their lives and be valued. We all must learn from the research and material presented here in order to fulfil these aims.

Ipswich, United Kingdom   Ellie Lindsay
                                        Lindsay Leg Club Foundation

Foreword II

Psychology and wounds: what, I ask rhetorically, connects these two apparently disparate subjects? Psychology is to me as a biomedical scientist, a subject which still strives for recognition as a true 'science', a subject not yet entirely based on empiricism. However, having closely studied wounds and their care for many years, this subject too is paradoxical. The cellular, biochemical and physiological aspects of wounding and healing are undoubtedly scientific in every sense of the word. The overwhelming research focus on wounds has thus far been directed at pathophysiology, healing mechanisms and treatments. Yet approaches to healing include a 'mystic' or 'art' component. I accept that my comments may cause some consternation amongst psychologists and wound clinicians alike!

Professor Upton and Dr have entitled his book *Psychology of Wounds and Wound Care in Clinical Practice*. It is all aspects of wounding, intrinsic and extrinsic, to which psychology applies. The circumstances leading up to an accident and traumatic wounding, patient self-neglect, mental health issues and self-harming – all have a psychology component.

Then there is the psychology of wound 'care': to explore this more closely, it is first necessary to delineate and define 'wound care' in greater detail. As I write this in June 2014, echoes of the Great war 1914–1918 reverberate loudly. This awful period was notable for death and wounds. War has been historically a time for great medical advances, not least in surgery and wound care. Countless amputees and disfigured troops returning from Europe were left in most cases to fend for themselves. In the Second World War we saw burned airmen treated by plastic surgeon Archie McIndoe, the 'guinea pigs' with terrible facial disfigurement. Such trauma accounts for more than skin and flesh wounds. Integral to such disfigurements, and the repeated surgery required to 'correct' deficits, is the adaptation to life thereafter and all that this entails. Indeed, post-treatment and the lifestyle sequelae of the wound patient have now become a matter of public interest and justifiably so.

This being the case, war wounds of the flesh demand the psychologist's attention as they are invariably associated to some degree with 'wounds' of the mind. Recent tragic events in Iraq and Afghanistan have similarly resulted in wounds to Western military personnel, with the attendant psychological trauma.

The majority of wounds are, however, of peacetime origin. Traumatic wounds such as burns are an unfortunate reality of life in all societies, bringing with them life-changing disfigurement in some cases. A personal interest, the so-called chronic wound similarly impacts on lifestyle. There are psychological issues linked with the aetiology and development of the chronic wounds; for example, the risks of non-compliance to treatment in 'lifestyle' diseases such as type 2 diabetes, the wilful ignorance of medical advice on diet and smoking, all play an important part in the prodromal phase of the relevant pathology. Which factors play a part in life with the wound, for the cosmetically altered patient, what influences beyond medicine influence recurrence?

In our aging population in the developed world, vascular disease, cancers and diabetes are having a huge impact on healthcare systems and on patients. The relatively recent attention paid to Quality of Life (QoL) reflects the progress of civilisation in this respect: an acknowledgement that wounds can, and do, impact on the everyday aspects of living for the patient and their families. Furthermore QoL can be empirically measured! Psychological science incorporated into the psychology of wound care.

Professor Upton is a prolific writer on matters of psychology in healthcare. We have been colleagues at Worcester where he initiated research into the patient experience of wound-related disease and of the hitherto neglected area of wound-related pain. Numerous articles now exist in the literature, providing the scientific foundation for this book. Such is the nature of this field of study, and of the consequences of wounds on society that I have no doubt this book will be followed by many others in the years to come!

Worcester, UK   Richard White

Preface

Chronic wounds have been described as: *"a silent epidemic that affects a large fraction of the world population and poses a major and gathering threat to the public health and economy"* (Sen et al. 2009, p.763) with over a quarter of a million people with chronic wounds in the UK and considerably more with acute wounds. The cost of these chronic wounds to the NHS in the UK has been estimated at £2–3 billion, approximately 3 % of NHS budget, with the additional cost of treating chronic wound patients for mood disorder estimated at being in the range of an additional £85.5 million to £100 million per annum (Upton and Hender 2012).

However, the impact is not just financial – it is something far more important than mere pounds, dollars or Euros – the psychosocial impact can be considerable. The psychological consequences of living with a chronic wound can include stress, anxiety, concerns about physical symptoms, low self-worth and feelings of despair. These can vary in severity, from minor negative emotions to suicidal thoughts, depending on each individual case (Upton and South 2011; Upton et al. 2012a, b, c).

Furthermore, the physiological effects of psychological concepts such as pain, stress and anxiety may result in delayed healing (Kiecolt-Glaser et al. 1995; Ebrecht et al. 2004; Upton 2011a, b; Woo 2010), prolonging suffering and treatment. This pain and stress may originate in the wound, the wound-dressing regimen or in the relationship the patient may have with their clinician. Psychological factors can prolong wound treatment by delaying healing and thereby increasing mood disorders, decreasing quality of life and increasing treatment costs. It is clear, therefore, that the psychological consequences of wounds are severe and that the psychological components of wound care are significant. This text seeks to address these two linked issues in one up-to-date book and, building on contemporary research evidence, present practical clinical guidelines for all clinicians involved in wound care.

The role of psychology in nursing and medical practice has become ever more significant in recent years, and this is reflected in various policy documents, educational developments and practice focus. Similarly, research exploring the role of psychology in wounds and wound care has grown considerably. For example, the role of stress on wound healing has developed since the 1980s, the impact of wounds on quality of life since the 1990s and the role of psychology in pain and pain management in wound care since the early 2000s (see Fig. 1).

This research, much of it practice focused, continues to grow in both scope and significance. This book is an attempt to synthesis some of this material and present contemporary evidence for the practicing clinician – whether they be a (specialist) nurse, a medic, podiatrist or any one of the myriad other professions associated with wound care today. I hope that you will be able

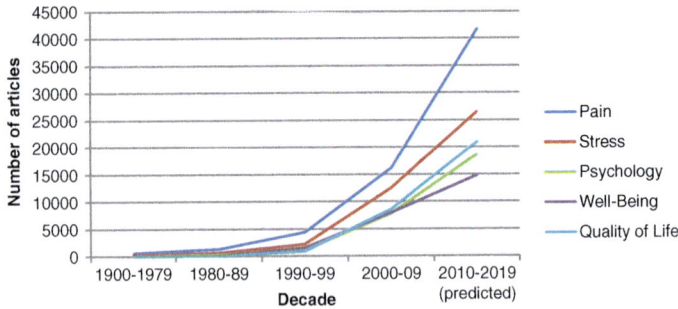

Figure 1 Number of articles published on psychology topics in wound care by decade

to use the material and the knowledge developed from this text within your practice for your clients' and patients' benefit.

This substantial body of literature has formed the backdrop of this book. Many (or perhaps in reality, *some*) of these publications have been read and presented here. Where some were more research focused, the key points have been distilled and presented for clinical practice. In short, this is a book that is academic in tone and presentation and also useful and relevant for practitioners from all backgrounds. In this way this text is inclusive in nature and demonstrates the importance of psychology in wound care today. We are passionate about psychology and, importantly, communicating its relevance and effectiveness in clinical practice. We hope that this comes through.

The aim of the text was, therefore, to demonstrate the value of psychology in wound care. Therefore, we have tried in this book to cover psychological aspects and concepts that have a direct role in this arena. However, this text does not claim to be comprehensive – it does not cover every single aspect of psychology, for this would be impossible; it does not even cover every single aspect of psychology related to wound care, as this too would be impossible. However, what has been achieved is a text that highlights the key areas in psychology related to wound care. Every chapter has been honed to ensure that every element is related to your current or future practice. Similarly, the whole feel of the text has been developed with key principles in mind:

- ***Contemporary research based evidence***: The book is based on contemporary research evidence to ensure that the guidance provided is rigorous and appropriate.
- ***Implications for practice***: The evidence and research material presented is related to clinical practice throughout.
- ***Concise and focused***: The material is presented in a clear, concise and focused manner to ensure readability by the busy professional.
- ***Academic but accessible***: We hope the writing is clear but academically robust in approach and presentation.

Structure of This Book

This book contains nine relatively short chapters that will engage you every step of the way to ensure you have contemporary and relevant information on the psychological aspects of wounds and wound care.

The book starts with Chap. 1 (where better to start), which explores the psychosocial aspects of living with wounds. For many years it has been recognised that chronic wounds come with a range of concomitant psychosocial issues. These may be related to the physiological aspects of the wound, or the reactions to these. Consequently, it is important to place these on record at the outset because these can be fundamental to understanding the psychological underpinnings and consequences described later in this text. Hence, this chapter will:

- Describe factors affecting people with wounds (e.g. the psychological impact of odour, exudate and the burden of having a chronic wound)
- Outline common psychological effects of wounds (e.g. emotional responses to appearance and body image issues)
- Outline how these factors can influence social functioning and psychological reactions

Chapter 2 will explore pain – one of the key elements facing those with wounds. The pain experienced during wound care can have a significant impact on the patient and on their treatment outcomes. Despite this, research shows that pain is not often assessed and therefore not adequately managed. This chapter aims to:

- Outline models of pain
- Explore levels of pain in those with wounds
- Outline how pain can be assessed and managed in wound care

Chapter 3 will explore a related topic – that of stress. Research has indicated a link between pain, stress and wound healing. It is essential therefore to ensure an adequate understanding of stress and how best to assess and manage it during any treatment regime. This chapter will:

- Explore models of stress and their relationship to wound care
- Highlight the relationship between stress and delayed healing
- Describe methods of assessing and managing stress

Research has shown that pain and stress of wound care can significantly impair quality of life and well-being. Additionally, quality of life and well-being can be greatly affected by other issues associated with wounds, which will be described in more detail in Chap. 4. This chapter aims to:

- Describe the concepts of quality of life and well-being and make important distinctions between the two
- Explore factors which impact on quality of life and well-being
- Discuss ways of measuring the two

There are a number of different types of wound, including diabetic foot ulcers, venous leg ulcers, traumatic wounds, pressure ulcers, surgical wounds, and burns. Important differences exist between these types of wound in terms of the psychological impact that they have on the individual and Chap. 5 aims to explore these. Specifically this chapter aims to:

- Explore how different types of wound have different psychological consequences
- Describe psychological issues for the patient with burns, diabetic foot ulcer, venous leg ulcers and pressure ulcers (e.g. pain levels and self-care)
- Use the variety of wounds types to exemplify the substantial role of psychology in wound care

In addition to the psychological consequences of the wounds themselves, research has shown that the treatment a patient receives can also have a significant impact on the individual and this will be the focus of Chap. 6. This chapter aims to:

- Provide an overview of the different treatments available (e.g. dressings, compression bandaging, negative pressure wound therapy)
- Explore the psychology of different forms of wound treatment
- Explore the psychological methods involved in dressing change and how material presented in previous chapters can be applied to dressing change

Chapter 7 aims to draw on areas highlighted in previous chapters (e.g. pain, stress, and psychological effects of wounds and treatment) to consider treatment concordance in people with wounds. Studies have also indicated that the relationship between patient and clinician may be of critical importance in treatment concordance. Hence, this chapter aims to:

- Describe factors affecting treatment concordance (including self-care)
- Consider the role of the health care professional in promoting concordance
- Identify factors which are important to patients, in terms of well-being and concordance

In Chap. 8, we will explore the research linking health and social support (including both formal and informal networks) since it has been identified as a key factor in the wound literature, indicating that social support can be particularly beneficial to people with wounds. This chapter aims to:

- Explore the concept of social support
- Explore the relationship between social support and well-being
- Consider the psychological impact of wounds on the individual's family/carers

The final chapter, Chap. 9, aims to bring together the issues described in the previous chapters and highlight the key messages which underpin the psychology of wound care. Specifically, this chapter aims to:

- Provide a summary of psychological issues in wound care
- Outline the key implications for practice
- Consider areas for future research
- Provide the patient voice

We hope that you will find this book useful and understand the relevance of psychology to your practice and thereby improve both the outcome and psychological health of all your patients.

References

Ebrecht M, Hextall J, Kirtley LG, Taylor A, Dyson M, Weinman J. Perceived stress and cortisol levels predict speed of wound healing in healthy male adults. Psychoneuroendocrinology. 2004;29(6):798–809.

Kiecolt-Glaser JK, Marucha PT, Malarkey WB, Mercado AM, Glaser R. Slowing of wound healing by psychological stress. Lancet. 1995;346:1194–6.

Sen CK, Gordillo GM, Roy S, Kirsner R, Lambert L, Hunt TK, Longaker MT. Human skin wounds: a major and snowballing threat to public health and the economy. Wound Repair Regen. 2009;17(6):763–71.

Upton D, Hender C. The Cost of Mood Disorder in Patients with Chronic Wounds. Wounds UK, 2012:8(1);107–109.

Upton D. Psychological impact of pain in patients with wounds. London: Wounds UK; 2011a.

Upton D. Psychology of stress. In: Upton D, editor. Psychological impact of pain in patients with wounds. London: Wounds UK; 2011b.

Upton D, South F. The psychological consequences of wounds – a vicious circle that should not be overlooked, Wounds UK. 2011;7(4):136–8.

Upton D, Hender C, Solowiej K. Mood disorders in patients with acute and chronic wounds: a health professional perspective. J Wound Care. 2012a;21(1):42–8.

Upton D, Hender C, Solowiej K, Woo K. Stress and pain associated with dressing change in chronic wound patients. J Wound Care. 2012b;22(2):53–61.

Upton D, Solowiej K, Hender C, Woodyat KY. Stress and pain associated with dressing change in patients with chronic wounds. J Wound Care. 2012c;21(2):53–61.

Woo KY. Wound-related pain: anxiety, stress and wound healing, Wounds UK. 2010;6(4):92–8.

Acknowledgements

Both of us have spent considerable time on this project, collating, reading and reviewing research articles and textbooks before trying to develop the material into a series of practical chapters that could assist and develop an individual professional's practice, whether they be psychologists, nurses, medics or other professions supporting those individuals with a wound. We have tried to encompass the literature from both an academic and a practitioner basis. We thank the researchers, clinicians and policy makers for all this work and the contributions they have made to the current knowledge base.

We must also offer thanks and acknowledgements to those who have provided support for us both at work and at home. We also thank our colleagues (for DU) at the University of Canberra and (for PU) at the University of Worcester for their help, advice, friendship and practical guidance.

In particular we would like to thank the following colleagues for their help in collating material for this book: Danni Stephens, Charlotte Makuire, Martha Jo Merrell, Abbye Andrews, and Lee Badham.

Finally, we would like to thank our family and friends for their continued support and patience. In particular, our children: Francesca, Rosie and Gabriel (all favourites).

Contents

1 **Psychosocial Consequences of Wounds** 1
   Summary 2
   Introduction 2
   Limitations of Daily Living. 4
   Social Isolation 5
   Disrupted Body Image/Sense of Self. 6
   Emotional Response 7
   Changes in Health Behaviours. 8
   Implications for Healing 9
   Psychological Resources 13
   Implications for Practice 15
   Conclusion 18
   References 18

2 **Pain** 25
   Summary 25
   Introduction 26
   Defining Pain 27
   Models of Pain 32
   Factors Influencing Pain 36
   Psychological Influences, Pain and Stress 38
   Assessing Pain 39
      Verbal Pain Rating Scale (VPRS)/Numerical
      Pain Rating Scale (NPRS) 40
      Visual Analogue Scale (VAS). 43
      The McGill Pain Questionnaire
      (MPQ; Melzack and Wall 1996) 43
      The Faces Pain Scale (Hockenberry et al. 2005). . . 43

	Pain Management	44
	Preparation	44
	Assessment	45
	Intervention	46
	Normalisation	50
	Summary	51
	References	51
3	**Stress**	**57**
	Summary	57
	Introduction	58
	General Adaption Syndrome (GAS) Model of Stress	60
	Interactional Model of Stress	63
	Assessing Stress	66
	The Perceived Stress Scale (PSS; Cohen 1983)	69
	The State Trait Anxiety Inventory (STAI; Speilberger 1977)	70
	The General Health Questionnaire (GHQ; Goldberg et al. 1978)	70
	The Hospital Anxiety and Depression Scale (HADS; Zigmond and Snaith 1983)	70
	Relationship Between Stress, Pain and Wound Healing	73
	Stress Management	77
	Managing Stressors	78
	Conclusion	80
	References	80
4	**Quality of Life and Well-Being**	**85**
	Summary	86
	Introduction	86
	Theories of QoL and Wellbeing	88
	Measuring Quality of Life	93
	Measuring Well-Being	98
	Factors Which Impact on Quality of Life and Well-Being	101
	Implications for Clinical Practice	103
	Conclusion	106
	References	107

5 Different Wound Type ... 113
- Summary ... 114
- Introduction ... 114
- Burns ... 115
- Diabetic Foot Ulcer (DFU) ... 123
- Venous Leg Ulcers ... 128
- Pressure Ulcers ... 131
- References ... 135

6 Treatment ... 143
- Summary ... 144
- Introduction ... 144
- Dressing Change ... 145
- Compression Bandaging ... 149
- Negative Pressure Wound Therapy ... 155
- Conclusion ... 161
- References ... 162

7 Concordance ... 167
- Summary ... 168
- Introduction ... 169
- Defining the Terms Compliance, Adherence and Concordance ... 170
- Models of Concordance ... 173
- Health Beliefs, Self-Regulation and Illness Perception ... 176
- Social Support ... 179
- Patient Satisfaction and Patient Centred Care ... 181
- Implications for Practice ... 184
- Conclusion ... 185
- References ... 186

8 Family, Friends and Social Support ... 191
- Summary ... 192
- Introduction ... 192
- What Is Social Support? ... 193
- How Does Social Support Protect Health? ... 196
- The Impact of Social Support on Health ... 199
- Social Support Interventions ... 202
- Family Considerations ... 205

Conclusion		209
References		210
9	**Conclusion**	217
	Summary	217
	Introduction	218
	Psychosocial Issues of Wounds	221
	Pain	223
	Stress	224
	Quality of Life and Well-Being	225
	Different Wound and Psychological Outcomes	227
	Different Treatments and Psychological Outcomes	228
	Communication and Concordance	230
	Family and Social Support	231
	Conclusion	232
	References	233
References		237
Index		241

Chapter 1
Psychosocial Consequences of Wounds

> Box 1.1: Key Points
> - A patient who is living with a chronic wound may experience a range of psychosocial consequences as a result of the wound and its treatment;
> - Pain, issues with mobility and treatment restrictions can result in limitations of daily activities such as general household tasks, maintenance of personal hygiene, and employment;
> - Social isolation may result from an inability to engage in social activities, a lack of energy resulting from sleep deprivation and the impact of emotional responses such as depression, anxiety, and embarrassment about wound malodour and leakage of exudate;
> - Women in particular may experience a disrupted body image and problems with self identity due to a perceived loss of femininity;
> - Emotional distress including depression, anxiety and stress are common responses to living with a chronic wound and its treatment;

- Psychological distress of living can provoke an increase in risky health behaviours such as smoking and alcohol consumption;
- A significant, negative relationship has been found between these psychosocial problems and the healing process;
- The relationship between psychosocial and physical health underlines the importance of taking a holistic approach to clinical care, rather than simply focusing on the physical signs and symptoms of the wound.

Summary

Patient centred practice, which focuses on an individual's illness experiences, not just on the clinical signs and symptoms of their wounds is essential. In recent years there has been a substantial increase in the range and scope of research addressing the psychosocial issues related to wound care, resulting in better understanding of the impact these can have both on the healing process, and a patient's wider quality of life (see Box 1.1). It is therefore essential that these issues be addressed in clinical practice. This chapter provides an overview of the psychosocial factors which are the focus of this book. The consequences for healing are summarized and the implications for clinical practice reviewed.

Introduction

A number of psychological consequences have been noted to occur for individuals living with wounds. These issues can be both specific (attached to a particular type of wound- see Chap. 5) and generic. For example, due to the complex nature of different wounds, the psychological effects of each can differ substantially. As is discussed in more detail in Chap. 5, wounds can be acute or chronic, which, along with the type (e.g. venous leg ulcer, pressure ulcer or burn) and site of the wound will have different implications for pain (Chap. 2) and stress (Chap. 3). This is also true in regard to the broader psychosocial impact of having a wound. Thus a patient's experience will differ depending on whether their wound is a chronic, persistent wound such as a venous leg ulcer or a diabetic foot ulcer for instance, or a trauma related wound such as that resulting from a burn or a surgical procedure.

Such psychological consequences can result from the wound itself, pain experienced from the wound and other physical consequences For example, it has been found that the common symptoms of chronic wounds – malodour and exudate – can increase negative emotions such as anxiety and depression (Hareendran et al. 2005; Herber et al. 2007). Furthermore many of the social implications of living with a wound can further exacerbate psychological health problems. Patients with exudate leakage and malodour often feel embarrassed, experiencing difficulty in maintaining outward appearance and dignity (Hyde et al. 1999; Walshe 1995). Such experiences can in turn lead to patients adopting maladaptive coping strategies, which can sometimes lead to the worsening of wounds (Lo et al. 2008). Such strategies might include the limiting of fluid intake in the hope of reducing exudate production, covering wounds to avoid leakage, and removing bandages in order to disperse exudate. Such experiences of exudate and malodour can also result in changes to a patient's appearance and choices of clothing and footwear (Persoon et al. 2004). This can also cause patients to feel embarrassment and negative body image (Herber et al. 2007), which causes them to retreat from social activities and contact with others, resulting in social isolation (Jones et al. 2008). Moreover this can lead in turn to a reduction in a patient's quality of life (Chap. 4). Thus we can see a cycle of physical problems and psychosocial difficulties which can ultimately delay the healing process (Fig. 1.1). This chapter provides an overview of the main psychosocial consequences of living

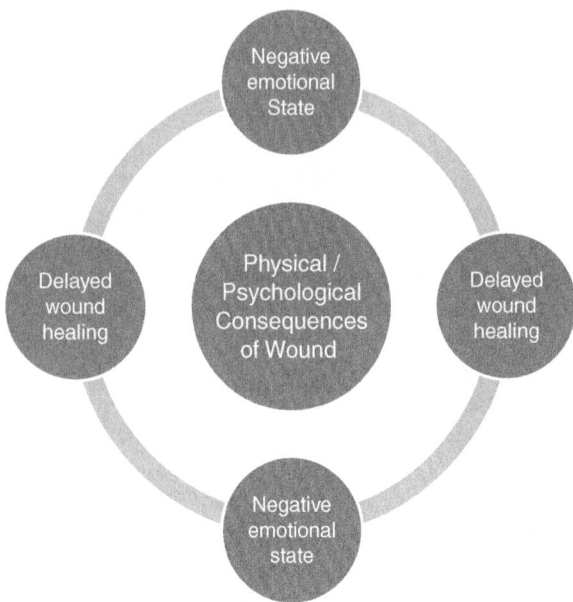

Figure 1.1 Psychological consequences of wounds

with a wound, and considers briefly how clinicians might best respond to these problems.

Limitations of Daily Living

Patients with chronic wounds often report feeling that they can no longer carry on with their daily routine and going out in public (Woo et al. 2009). Furthermore, patients may have to limit their activities in order to reduce painful experiences (Woo 2010), subsequently reducing their social mobility (Solowiej et al. 2010a). Herber et al. (2007) discovered that patients will often avoid activities such as walking, shopping and exercising, due the pain attributed to such activities. In addition to this, patients have also reported avoiding these activities due to worries that they will lead to, or contribute, to further wound-related difficulties (Persoon et al. 2004). Thus patients with chronic wounds may experience quite severe restriction in the daily activities we often take for granted because of pain and limitations of movement. Impaired mobility can also lead to the inability to work (Faria et al. 2011), perform general household tasks (Woo et al. 2009) and maintain personal hygiene (Fox 2002). Such restrictions can have significant implications for a patient's psychological health, and patients often believe them to be one of the worse aspects of having a wound (Hamer et al. 1994). As such, it is possible for a negative cyclical relationship to occur, whereby the negative consequences of the wound result in a negative emotional state, impacting upon wound healing and, subsequently, leading to further negative emotions (See Fig. 1.1).

Social Isolation

These limitations in daily activities often result in individuals becoming increasingly isolated from others (Gorecki et al. 2009). Exclusion from social activities has also been related to the intrusion of treatment – either because of the need to attend clinic, or wait in for a nursing visit (Hopkins 2004a, b). In addition it has been found that patients will limit their involvement in leisure activities such as swimming, gardening, walking and travelling (Krasner 1998; Chase et al. 2000; Hareendran et al. 2005) which then results in reduced social contact. For example, Hamer et al. (1994) found that almost half of the patients they spoke to had given up some of their hobbies. This reduction in social activities and interactions with others may also stem from a lack of energy, caused by the sleep deprivation that can result from the intense pain of a chronic wound (Harlin et al. 2009; Upton and Andrews 2013a, b, c). Furthermore, the feelings of helplessness and anxiety associated with not being able to continue with daily activities can contribute further to social isolation and feelings of disconnection from society (Brown 2005a, b, c).

Anxiety is not the only emotional response that may contribute to a patient withdrawing from interactions with others. The relationship between depression and social withdrawal has long been recognised (Baddeley et al. 2013); thus the depression associated with having a chronic wound may well change social relationships. Furthermore, a spiral relationship may well develop in which depression leads to withdrawal from social interaction leading in turn to increased dysphoria (Hawkley and Cacioppo 2003). Embarrassment has also been highlighted as a reason for social withdrawal in this group. This has been linked in particular to the unpleasant odour, which can often accompanies a chronic wound. Concerns about whether others can detect this malodour can lead to patients trying to keep themselves safe from the scrutiny of others, and the possibility of undesirable comments about their cleanliness (Probst et al. 2013). Furthermore, reduced personal hygiene can be a genuine concern; patients may avoid washing for fear that dressings might get wet and that this will disrupt the healing process (Douglas 2001; Ebbeskog and Ekman 2001a, b). Thus withdrawal from society can result from embarrassment over these changes in levels of personal care as well as the malodour of the wound itself.

Having a chronic wound may also change interpersonal relationships in other ways. Role reversal in families, where the previous head of the family becomes the dependent one, has been described (Douglas 2001; see Chap. 8). In intimate relationships for example, where a partner has to take on the role of carer, the dynamic may well change; furthermore, couples may experience a loss of physical and emotional intimacy (Gorecki et al. 2009).

Disrupted Body Image/Sense of Self

This change in the dynamics of intimate relationships may also result from a shift in the patient's self-perception and a loss of identity (Probst et al. 2013). Research has highlighted the impact of these issues on women in particular (Hyland et al. 1994). Compression bandages, wrapping, and other dressings can be bulky and may require a wardrobe adjustment and this can lead to a perceived loss of femininity for some women (Hyland et al. 1994). Feelings of shame, embarrassment, and diminished femininity have also been observed in women with malignant fungating wounds in progressive breast cancer (Boon et al. 2000). Given the significance of the female breast as a symbol of sexuality and femininity, learning that a wound in this area can impact on a woman's body image and self-concept is not surprising. Furthermore, symptoms such as malodour, an excess of exudate and relentless seepage, need constant vigilance and management when in public (for example having to carry additional changes of clothes). Such extreme changes in behaviour can contribute to the loss of sense of self and social identity (Probst et al. 2013). Moreover malodour and excessive exudate can also lead to feelings of disgust, self-loathing, and low self-esteem (Jones et al. 2008).

Emotional Response

The emotional reaction to having a chronic wound usually includes some form of distress –depression, anxiety and stress are common responses. For example, burn injuries have been linked to serious emotional difficulties including anxiety and post traumatic stress disorder (Van Loey and Van Son 2003; Loncar et al. 2006). Furthermore, research exploring the prevalence of depression and anxiety in 190 patients with chronic venous ulcerations, indicated that 27 % of patients were experiencing depression with 26 % being highly anxious (Jones et al. 2006). In a similar vein, Searle et al. (2005) found that following diagnosis with a foot ulcer, depressed mood was a very common response to a number of features of the wound including the time taken to heal, loss of independence, and the limitations of daily living. Changes in role and an increase in dependency on others can also trigger anxiety (Herber et al. 2007) and guilt (Walshe 1995). In addition, the visibility of the wound, including smell and leakage of exudate may also lead to feelings of vulnerability and embarrassment resulting in further anxiety and distress (Piggin and Jones 2007; Lo et al. 2008; Alexander, 2010). Treatment may also trigger feelings of distress: studies in patients with a range of different types of chronic wound have shown that stress and anxiety is linked to the pain of dressing change as well as the stress of background pain (Upton et al. 2013c; Upton et al. 2012b, c) Finally, the sleep disturbances which many experience because of wound pain can also lead to patients experiencing heightened worry and frustration – which further disrupts sleep; Cole-King and Harding (2001) and Fagervik-Morton and Price (2009) have discovered that anxiety and depression can also contribute to sleep disturbance.

Sleep deprivation, which is thought to impact on healing, has been found to be particularly prevalent in patients living with chronic wounds. Research suggests that approximately 25 % of patients experience at least three nights of sleep disturbance due to their wound, whilst 49 % of patients reported experiencing sleep disturbance due to their wound on six or more nights (Price and Harding 1993). Upton and Andrews (2013a, b, c) also reported on the sleep disturbance in those with chronic wounds, with their results suggesting a more significant issue than that Price and Harding (1993). Specifically, Sixty-nine per cent of their leg ulcer patients reported sleep disruption, with 88 % stating that they wake at least once during the night. General wound pain was the most frequently-cited cause (58 %), while pain associated with treatment affected the sleep of 38 % of respondents. Sleep disruption in people with chronic wounds is an important issue since it can impact on pain levels, wellbeing, quality of life and healing.

Changes in Health Behaviours

There is evidence that psychological distress can increase risky health behaviours such as smoking and alcohol consumption (Upton and Thirlaway 2014); thus individuals experiencing high levels of stress are more likely to increase their alcohol (Sillaber and Henniger 2004) and tobacco use (Sinha 2008). A link to depression, anxiety and social isolation has also been noted specifically in older adult drinkers (Schonfeld and Dupree 1991). Furthermore studies have identified a relationship between stress and increased participation in health damaging behaviours in individuals with chronic wounds (Gouin and Kiecolt-Glaser 2011). This is a concern because behaviours such as this have been shown to impede the healing process.

Implications for Healing

The psychosocial issues described so far in this chapter are important in part because of the implications they have for a patient's mental health and quality of life. However, this is not their only relevance. A significant, negative relationship has been found between these psychosocial problems and the healing process. Studies have demonstrated that patients who are anxious about their physical condition, or who feel depressed, tend to show much slower healing rates than patients with a more positive attitude. For example Doering et al. (2005) found that following surgery, patients with more depressive symptoms at discharge had more infections and poorer wound healing than patients who reported less distress. Likewise, Cole-King and Harding (2001) showed that patients with leg ulcers who experienced the highest levels of depression and anxiety were four times more likely to show delayed healing compared to individuals who reported less distress. Furthermore, distress predicted wound healing outcomes over and above differences in other variables such as demographic and medical status. Research exploring mucosal wound healing and presentation of dysphoria has also provided support for this link. Bosch et al. (2007), examined the patients' levels of dysphoria and rate of wound healing, discovering that patients who presented with higher levels of dysphoria were approximately 3.6 times more likely to experience slower wound healing whilst also exhibiting larger wound sizes. Similar outcomes have also been demonstrated with patients suffering from burns (Wilson et al. 2011).

A wealth of research is also available which considers the relationship between a patient's perceived stress and the rate of wound healing (Cole-King and Harding 2001; Gouin and Kiecolt-Glaser 2011; Soon and Acton 2006; Woo 2010). This work has linked both wound pain and treatment pain with poorer patient outcomes. For example, Upton and colleagues have suggested a link between pain, stress and healing in those with a chronic wound (e.g. Upton 2011a; Solowiej et al. 2009, 2010a, b). In particular, the evidence they present suggests that the stress of dressing change can be a significant factor in those with a chronic wound. Stress is thought to influence healing partly through its impact on immune functioning; stress reduces the levels of the many inflammatory cytokines and enzymes that are necessary for tissue repair (Upton 2011a) and increases levels of cortisol. In addition to this physiological response, patients may have a behavioural response to stress which impacts on healing. It has been suggested that stress increases the likelihood of patients making poor cognitive judgments such as avoiding treatment because dressing removal is perceived as an unpleasant experience. Thus negative emotional responses affect biological and behavioural responses resulting in delayed wound healing. The relationship between pain, stress and wound healing is therefore both statistically significant and clinically relevant (Gouin and Kiecolt-Glaser 2010; Upton et al. 2012a, b, c).

Sleep deprivation is also detrimental to the healing process. As noted earlier, sleep disturbances are often associated with the onset of psychological distress and with the pain accompanying with living with a wound. This has significant implications for wound healing since even mild sleep deprivation has been shown to impair immune functioning (Kahan et al. 2010; Harlin et al. 2009). For example, just one night of sleep deprivation has been discovered to impact wound healing (Altemus et al. 2001). It is thought that sleep disturbance, like stress, reduces cytokin levels and alters killer cell activity, subsequently slowing skin barrier repair (Altemus et al. 2001).

Changes in behaviour such as smoking, alcohol consumption, poor diet and lack of exercise are also thought to impact on healing. Research has shown that surgical patients who are considered regular smokers have significantly slower healing periods that those classed as non-smokers (Silverstein 1992). This is thought to be because the toxins and nicotine within cigarette smoke reduce oxygen levels in the blood whilst also reducing macrophage function (Silverstein 1992). Given the known link between hypoxia and reduced healing (Gordillo and Sen 2003), this relationship is not suprsing. The negative implications of smoking for wound healing are further illustrated by research exploring smoking cessation programmes (Moller et al. 2002): implementation of such programmes 6–8 weeks before scheduled surgery has been found to reduce post-surgical wound complications. Similarly, alcohol consumption has been linked to slower healing (Benveniste and Thut 1981). Animal studies have highlighted the effects of alcohol use, demonstrating the disruption to numerous mechanisms which underpin the healing process. For example, alcohol use before or after wounding can impair the inflammatory response that is essential in the initial healing stages (Fitzgerald et al. 2007). Animal studies have also shown that heavy alcohol use is associated with delays in cell migration and collagen deposition at the wound site, which in turn can impede the healing process (Benveniste and Thut 1981). A link between preoperative alcohol use and postoperative morbidity has also been shown in humans (Tønnesen and Kehlet 1999). Finally diet and exercise have also been linked to the rate of wound healing. For example, nutritional deficits including, low protein, low glucose intake and vitamin deficiencies, can all impede the wound healing process (Russell 2001; Posthauer 2006; McDaniel et al. 2008). Lack of regular physical activity has also been shown to slow wound healing rate in animal models (Keylock et al. 2008). Furthermore, studies with human patients have shown that regular exercise can lead to reduced wound healing time

(Upton 2011a, b). For example, whilst it was found that a 3-day exercise programme did not positively impact wound healing (Altemus et al. 2001), research implementing a 4 week programme resulted in a 25 % improvement in punch biopsy wound healing (Emery et al. 2005).

As described earlier, the experience of living with a chronic wound brings with it a number of factors (e.g. malodour, exudate, restricted mobility, aspects of treatment) which can lead to a patient reducing their participation in social activities, often becoming isolated. When an individual withdraws from social interactions, they forsake an important aspect of psychosocial support. Thus there is a whole range of practical and emotional support which is no longer accessible to an individual. As social support has been found to be important for emotional wellbeing and quality of life, acting as a buffer against stress and enhancing physical health (Thoits 2011) this has implications for wound healing. The evidence from clinical populations suggests that social isolation has an indirect effect on wound healing because of the impact it has on our emotional health which was noted earlier (Hawkley and Cacioppo 2003); this increased distress further hinders healing by reducing inflammatory cytokines and increasing cortisol concentrations as already described. However, animal studies have identified a more direct pathway for this influence. Detillion et al. (2004) found that stress did increase cortisol concentrations, thereby impairing wound healing in hamsters, but only in those animals that were kept in isolation. Socially housed animals did not show this effect. Furthermore, isolated hamsters that had been given an adrenalectomy, and therefore could not produce cortisol, did not show delayed wound healing. In contrast treating isolated hamsters with the hormone oxytocin, which is released during social contact, blocked stress-induced increases in cortisol, and wound healing was facilitated. This suggests that social isolation increases stress-related cortisol production thereby slowing wound healing. Whilst studies with human populations show inconsistent effects for oxytocin in social behaviours, it seems increasingly likely that this is because the oxytocin mechanism is controlled to some extent by social contexts and individual differences (Bartz, et al. 2011);

such differences may include factors such as personality and psychological resources.

Psychological Resources

Psychological resources refer to emotional and cognitive factors such as optimism, personal control, social support and active coping all of which are known to be protective of mental health (Taylor et al. 2000). Moreover there is evidence that the presence of these positive features may also foster good physical health (DeLongis et al. 1988; Schöllgen et al. 2011). Thus the presence of positive psychological resources may act as a buffer against the impact of the negative aspects of ill health. For example, individuals who seek information or advice about their wound and its treatment may find this gives them greater personal control of their health and also decreases feelings of distress (Moffatt et al. 2011). The significance of this personal control for enabling individuals to live well with a chronic wound is demonstrated very clearly by Probst et al. (2013), who looked at the experience of women with fungating wounds. In this study, some of the women had been through a very personal process of working out what adjustments they needed to make to their lives in order to manage their condition so as to enable them to continue to live a normal life – going to work, seeing friends and so on. These women seemed to have accepted the situation and the changes they had had to make to accommodate the person they had become. This self-efficacy – the belief that you can do something – gave them the ability to adjust to their new identity, taking control of the situation, and furthermore, insisting that everyone else (including intimate partners) also accept this new reality.

The women in Probst et al.'s study, showed what has been termed resilience – they had successfully adapted in order to maintain (or regain) their emotional well-being in the face of adversity (Trivedi et al. 2011). Traditionally resilience (also sometimes referred to as hardiness) has been linked to the coping that is seen in some individuals following traumatic events, disasters or personal tragedy. This model sees resilience as an intrinsic ability, which prevents the typical distress response to stressful events. Thus resilience is a personality trait, which protects people from stress. However, there is increasing recognition of the role that resilience might play in chronic illness (Trivedi et al. 2011). This view conceptualises resilience as a resource which allows us to recover more quickly from stressful events or illness experiences. Thus rather than seeing resilient individuals as those who have immunity to illness, this approach accepts that everyone, even resilient individuals, will experience transitory distress during a stressful event such as diagnosis of chronic illness. The difference between the resilient and the vulnerable individual, is that the resilient person will make a speedy recovery, whilst the vulnerable one may maintain a position of stress. If we accept this definition of resilience – that it is an attribute which aids speedy recovery – then resilience becomes something that can be moderated in order improve patient outcomes.

Resilience has been linked to another personality trait – optimism. Optimism provides a predisposition to expect positive outcomes. This is a trait which has been linked to faster recovery from acute illness episodes such as heart surgery (Scheier et al. 1999) and better coping in longer term problems such as breast cancer (Carver, et al. 1993). It has also been linked to conscientiousness, which is defined as the tendency to act dutifully, be self-disciplined and to aim for achievement (McCrae and John 1992). Conscientiousness has also been associated with longer survival in the chronically ill (Christensen et al. 2012). Furthermore, there is evidence that resilience is enhanced by social relationships.

This link between resilience and social support may provide the mechanism by which to moderate resilience, since social support – the presence of caring supportive relationships – has been found to foster positive outcomes in a number of chronic illnesses. Searle and colleagues (2005) found for example that interacting with other patients provided a good source of social support; sharing personal experiences of living with diabetes, provided patients with a sense of camaraderie and identity. There is evidence that from case studies (e.g. Lindsay 2013; Shuter et al. 2011) those patients with seemingly intractable leg wounds heal once they start attending support groups within the community. Known as a 'leg club', these interventions aim to improve an individual's well-being. Some well-known programmes include 'Lively legs' programme (Heinen et al. 2012); 'Look after your legs' support group (Freeman et al. 2007); and the 'Lindsay leg club' ® (Lindsay 2013). It may well be that these groups are effective because they are able to promote resilience, and provide the right context for physiological features of healing, such as the oxytocin mechanism, to be activated (more discussion on social support and such Leg Clubs are presented in Chap. 8).

Implications for Practice

Modern wound care practices include many advanced techniques, yet despite these there are patients with chronic, complex wounds that do not heal (Vermeiden et al. 2009). It has been recognised that for these patients psychosocial factors play a significant role in the healing process (Guo and DiPietro 2010). However, there is evidence that in daily practice, little attention is paid to these factors (Gorecki et al. 2009). There are three possible explanations for the neglect of psychosocial factors. Firstly, many clinicians admit that symptom control is usually the main nursing priority, (Naylor 2002). Secondly, clinicians may not always be aware of the patient's emotional response (Green and Jester 2009). For example Searle and colleagues (2005) found that podiatrists caring for patients with diabetic foot ulcers were often not aware of the patient's true feelings as patients were able to present a positive exterior in order to dissemble. Finally, it must be acknowledged that managing the psychological component of wound care can be challenging.

It has therefore been suggested that more translational work is needed to develop innovative treatments which have the power to reduce stress-induced delays in wound healing (Gouin and Kiecolt-Glaser 2010). Whilst this is undoubtedly true, there are already a number of things that the clinician can do to ensure that the psychosocial needs of their patients are given full consideration. Indeed, the attitude and approach of a healthcare professional can change the patient experience (Jester and Green 2009; see Chap. 7). Thus medical treatment delivered by an empathetic and compassionate clinician can enable the patient to have a more positive experience. Indeed, patients recognise the importance of the healthcare professional's crucial role in the treatment and management of wounds and are sensitive to inconsistency in care, information giving and negative attitudes (Spilsbury et al. 2007). Whilst a lack of consistency and compassion will have an adverse affect on the patient experience, good care from a specialist clinician reduces distress, embarrassment and social isolation (Lo et al. 2008).

Treatment for a chronic wound should always start with a comprehensive assessment that includes the evaluation of a patient's psychosocial concerns. This will allow the development of an appropriate individualized treatment plan that can include interventions to address the issues identified (Alexander 2013). If a team of health care professionals are to be involved in an individual's care, then it is essential that this treatment plan is shared by the team so as to ensure a consistent approach, as this is appreciated by patients, and reduces confusion and anxiety about the care being delivered (Spilsbury et al. 2007).

Providing accurate and honest information about the nature of the wound condition, the chosen treatment, and prognosis is also essential. Patients have reported frustration with evasive or inaccurate responses from clinicians about healing progress; whilst positive but untrue statements about progress in situations where recovery is delayed may be delivered with good intentions, honesty is far more effective in dispelling anxiety about the healing process. Being candid about set backs allows patients to have a realistic expectations of recovery. Furthermore, providing accurate individual assessment and information has been shown to increase patient compliance and change health behaviours in a positive way (Heinen et al. 2012). In contrast lack of information and practical help from health professionals can result in patients using poor management strategies that could harm their wound, aggravate problems such as bleeding and impair healing (Lo et al. 2008). In contrast, where recovery is slow, patients may experience frustration at the lack of progress and find it difficult to accept the assurances of the clinician that progress is being made. In such cases photography may provide an easy and effective method of offering accurate feedback to a patient during treatment: weekly photos can provide a concrete record of progress which allows the healing process to be more easily recognized by the patient. This might also be useful in cases where the wound is located in a site not easily accessible to the patient (e.g. pressure ulcers) meaning that they are totally dependent on others for information about progress with healing (Spilsbury et al. 2007).

Acknowledging and managing patient distress is also very important. Teaching a simple relaxation technique such as controlled breathing or guided imagery may help patients cope with stressful situations such as dressing change. Counselling or professional intervention may be indicated where patient distress has become severe, in particular where depression or anxiety has become significant. Alternatively patients may be supported to find their own coping mechanisms by finding new ways to deal with their situation. For example for patients whose customary leisure pursuits are no longer possible for practical reasons, encouraging them to find new interests may be one way of helping them to take an active approach to coping with their change in health status and identity. Furthermore engaging in enjoyable activities will support positive wellbeing.

Finally the importance of providing patients with a support network should not be neglected. Encouraging patients to maintain social activities and interactions with family and friends is obviously important. Furthermore, the clinician could focus on involving the family in the treatment where this is possible or desirable (Vermeiden et al. 2009). Finally the advantages of establishing support groups for patients and their carers have already been discussed in this chapter: not only do such groups enables the sharing of experiences and learning from others in a similar situation, by reducing social isolation they may well influence the physical healing process.

Conclusion

This chapter has demonstrated, albeit briefly, the importance of taking a holistic approach to wound care. A patient's emotional, social and psychological needs are as central to practice as their physical needs. The psychosocial factors explored include limitations to daily activities, stress, depression, anxiety, embarrassment, changes to self identity and social isolation. Many of these consequences stem from the physical aspects of having a chronic wound such as pain, exudate, malodour, restricted mobility, sleep disturbance and lack of energy. However focusing on simply treating the physical wound is likely to be ineffective, since psychosocial factors can impede the healing process. Furthermore, aspects of the treatment itself may exacerbate some of these psychosocial features. In addition, maladaptive changes in behaviour may result from reduced psychosocial health, including poor eating habits and increased smoking and drinking, all of which are known to impair healing and may also increase wound severity. It is therefore not unexpected that patients with wounds have a significantly poorer quality of life compared to the general population. From a clinical perspective, it is therefore important to recognise psychological and social aspects of living with a chronic wound, and to develop comprehensive approaches to care that prioritise the needs of the individual patient in order to ensure that wound care is optimised.

References

Alexander SJ. Time to get serious about assessing–and managing–psychosocial issues associated with chronic wounds. Curr Opin Support Palliat Care. 2013;7(1):95–100.

Altemus M, Rao B, Dhabhar FS, Ding W, Granstein RD. Stress-induced changes in skin barrier function in healthy women. J Invest Dermatol. 2001;117(2):309–17.

Baddeley JL, Pennebaker JW, Beevers CG. Everyday social behavior during a major depressive episode. Soc Psychol Pers Sci. 2013;4(4): 445–52.

Bartz JA, Zaki J, Bolger N, Ochsner KN. Social effects of oxytocin in humans: context and person matter. Trends Cogn Sci. 2011;15(7): 301–9.

Benveniste K, Thut P. The effect of chronic alcoholism on wound healing. Proc Soc Exp Biol Med. 1981;166:568–75.

Boon H, Brophy J, Lee J. The community care of a patient with a fungating wound. Br J Nurs. 2000;9(1 Suppl):S35–8.

Bosch JA, Engeland CG, Cacioppo JT, Marucha PT. Depressive symptoms predict mucosal wound healing. Psychosom Med. 2007;69:597–605.

Brown A. Chronic leg ulcers, part 1: do they affect a patient's social life? Br J Nurs. 2005a;14(17):894–8.

Brown A. Chronic leg ulcers, part 2: do they affect a patient's social life? Br J Nurs. 2005b;14(18):986–9.

Brown G. Speech to the volunteering conference, London, 2005c. 31 Jan 2005.

Carver CS, Pozo C, Harris SD, Noriega V, Scheier MF, Robinson DS, Clark KC. How coping mediates the effect of optimism on distress: a study of women with early stage breast cancer. J Pers Soc Psychol. 1993;65(2):375.

Chase SK, Whittemore R, Crosby N, Freney D, Howes P, Phillips TJ. Living with chronic venous ulcers: a descriptive study of knowledge and functional health status. J Community Health Nurs. 2000;17(1):1–13.

Christensen K, McGue M. Commentary: twins, worms and life course epidemiology. Int J Epidemiol. 2012;41(4):1010–1.

Cole-King A, Harding KG. Psychological factors and delayed healing in chronic wounds. Psychosom Med. 2001;63:216–20.

DeLongis A, Folkman S, Lazarus RS. The impact of daily stress on health and mood: psychological and social resources as mediators. J Pers Soc Psychol. 1988;54(3):486.

Detillion CE, Craft TK, Glasper ER, Prendergast BJ, DeVries AC. Social facilitation of wound healing. Psychoneuroendocrinology. 2004;29(8):1004–11.

Doering LV, Moser DK, Lemankiewicz W, et al. Depression, healing, and recovery from coronary artery bypass surgery. Am J Crit Care. 2005;14(4):316–24.

Douglas V. Living with a chronic leg ulcer: an insight into patients' experiences and feelings. J Wound Care. 2001;10(9):355–60.

Ebbeskog B, Ekman S-L. Elderly persons' experiences of living with venous leg ulcer: living in a dialectical relationship between freedom and imprisonment. Scand J Caring Sci. 2001a;235–243.

Ebbeskog B, Ekman S. Elderly people's experiences: the meaning of living with venous leg ulcer. Eur Wound Manag Assoc J. 2001b; 1(1):21–3.

Emery CF, Kiecolt-Glaser JK, Glaser R, Malarkey WB, Frid DJ. Exercise accelerates wound healing among healthy older adults: a preliminary investigation. J Gerontol A Biol Sci Med Sci. 2005;60(11):1432–6.

Fagervik-Morton H, Price P. Chronic ulcers and everyday living: patients' perspective in the United Kingdom. Wounds. 2009; 21(12):318–23.

Faria E, Blanes L, Hochman B, et al. Health-related quality of life, self-esteem, and functional status of patients with leg ulcers. Wounds. 2011;23(1):4–10.

Fitzgerald DJ, Radek KA, Chaar M, Faunce DE, DiPietro LA, Kovacs EJ. Effects of acute ethanol exposure on the early inflammatory response after excisional injury. Alcohol Clin Exp Res. 2007;31(2):317–23.

Fox C. Living with a pressure ulcer: a descriptive study of patients' experiences. Br J Community Nurs. 2002;7(6 Suppl):10–22.

Freeman E, Gibbins A, Walker M, Hapeshi J. 'Look after your legs': patients' experience of an assessment clinic. Br J Community Nurs. 2007;12(1 Suppl):S19–25.

Gordillo GM, Sen CK. Revisiting the essential role of oxygen in wound healing. Am J Surg. 2003;186(3):259–63.

Gorecki C, Brown JM, Nelson EA, Briggs M, Schoonhoven L, Dealey C, et al. Impact of pressure ulcers on quality of life in older patients: a systematic review. J Am Geriatr Soc. 2009; 57(7):1175–83.

Gouin JP, Kiecolt-Glaser JK. The impact of psychological stress on wound healing: methods and mechanisms. Immunol Allergy Clin North Am. 2011;31(1):81–93.

Green J, Jester R. Health-related quality of life and chronic venous leg ulceration: part 1. Wound Care. 2009;14(12):12–7.

Guo S, DiPietro LA. Factors affecting wound healing. J Dent Res. 2010;89(3):219–29.

Hamer C, Cullum N, Roe BH. Patients' perceptions of chronic leg ulcers. J Wound Care. 1994;3(2):99–101.

Hareendran A, Bradbury A, Budd J, Geroulakos G, Hobbs R, Kenkre J, Symonds T. Measuring the impact of venous leg ulcers on quality of life. J Wound Care. 2005;14(2):53–7.

Harlin SL, Harlin RD, Sherman TI, Rozsas CM, Shafqat SM, Meyers W. Using a structured, computer-administered questionnaire for evaluating health-related quality of life in patients with chronic lower extremity wounds. Ostomy Wound Manage. 2009;55(9): 30–9.

Hawkley LC, Cacioppo JT. Loneliness and pathways to disease. Brain Behav Immun. 2003;17(1):98–105.

Heinen M, Borm G, van der Vleuten C, Evers A, Oostendorp R, van Achterberg T. The lively legs self-management programme increased physical activity and reduced wound days in leg ulcer patients: results from a randomized controlled trial. Int J Nurs Stud. 2012;49:151–61.

Herber OR, Schnepp W, Rieger MA. A systematic review on the impact of leg ulceration on patients' quality of life. Health Qual Life Outcomes. 2007;5(44):1–12.

Hopkins A. Disrupted lives: investigating coping strategies for non-healing leg ulcers. Br J Nurs. 2004a;13(9):556–63.

Hopkins A. The use of qualitative research methodologies to explore leg ulceration. J Tissue Viability. 2004b;14(4):142–7.

Hyde C, Ward B, Horsfall J, Winder G. Older women's experience of living with chronic leg ulceration. Int J Nurs Pract. 1999;5: 189–98.

Hyland M. Quality of life of leg ulcer patients: questionnaire and preliminary findings. J Wound Care. 1994;3(6):294–8.

Jones J, Barr W, Robinson J, Carlisle C. Depression in patients with chronic venous ulceration. Br J Nurs. 2006;15(11):17–23.

Jones JE, Robinson J, Barr W, Carlisle C. Impact of exudate and odour from chronic venous leg ulceration. Nurs Stand. 2008; 22(45):53–61.

Kahan V, Ribeiro DA, Andersen ML, Alvarenga TA, Tufik S. Sleep loss induces differential response related to genotoxicity in multiple organs of three different mice strains. Basic Clin Pharmacol Toxicol. 2010;107:598–602. doi:10.1111/j.1742-7843.2010.00540.x.

Keylock KT, Vieira VJ, Wallig MA, et al. Exercise accelerates cutaneous wound healing and decreases wound inflammation in aged mice. Am J Physiol Regul Integr Comp Physiol. 2008;294(1):R179–84.

Krasner D. Painful venous ulcers: themes and stories about their impact on quality of life. Ostomy Wound Manage. 1998;44(9): 38–46.

Lindsay E. Changing policy and practice to empower older people living with chronic wounds. Symposium abstract; The 20th IAGG world congress of gerontology and geriatrics, Korea. 2013.

Lo SF, Hu WY, Hayter M, Chang SC, Hsu MY, Wu LY. Experiences of living with a malignant fungating wound: a qualitative study. J Clin Nurs. 2008;17(20):2699–708.

Loncar Z, Bras M, Mickovic V. The relationships between burn pain, anxiety and depression. Coll Antropol. 2006;30(2):319–25.

McCrae RR, John OP. An introduction to the five-factor model and its applications. J Pers. 1992;60(2):175–215.

McDaniel JC, Belury M, Ahijevych K, et al. Omega-3 fatty acids effect on wound healing. Wound Repair Regen. 2008;16(3): 337–45.

Moffatt CJ, Mapplebeck L, Murray S, Morgan P. The experience of patients with complex wounds and the use of NPWT in a home-care setting. J Wound Care. 2011;20(11):512.

Moller AM, Villebro N, Pedersen T, Tonnesen H. Effect of preoperative smoking intervention on postoperative complications: a randomised clinical trial. Lancet. 2002;359:114–7.

Naylor W. Malignant wounds: aetiology and principles of management. Nurs Stand. 2002;16(52):45–53.

Persoon A, Heinen M, van der Vleuten C, de Rooij M, van de Kerkhof P, van Achterberg T. Leg ulcers: a review of their impact on daily life. J Clin Nurs. 2004;13(3):341–54.

Piggin C, Jones V. Malignant fungating wounds: an analysis of the lived experience. Int J Palliat Care. 2007;13:384–91.

Posthauer ME. The role of nutrition in wound care. Adv Skin Wound Care. 2006;19(1):43–52.

Probst S, Arber A, Faithfull S. Malignant fungating wounds–the meaning of living in an unbounded body. Eur J Oncol Nurs. 2013;17(1):38–45.

Price P, Harding KG. Defining quality of life. J Wound Care. 1993;2:304–6.

Russell L. The importance of patients' nutritional status in wound healing. Br J Nurs. 2001;10(6 Suppl):S44–9. S42.

Schöllgen I, Huxhold O, Schüz B, Tesch-Römer C. Resources for health: differential effects of optimistic self-beliefs and social support according to socioeconomic status. Health Psychol. 2011; 30(3):326.

Schonfeld L, Dupree LW. Antecedents of drinking for early-and late-onset elderly alcohol abusers. J Stud Alcohol Drugs. 1991; 52(6):587.

Scheier MF, Matthews KA, Owens JF, Schulz R, Bridges MW, Magovern GJ, et al. Optimism and rehospitalization after coronary artery bypass graft surgery. Arch Intern Med. 1999;159:829–35.

Searle A, Campbell R, Tallon D, Fitzgerald A, Vedhara K. A qualitative approach to understanding the experience of ulceration and healing in the diabetic foot: patient and podiatrist perspectives. Wounds. 2005;17(1):16–26.

Shuter P, Finlayson K, Edwards H, Courtney M, Cheryl H, Lindsay E. Leg clubs – beyond the ulcers: case studies based on participatory action research. Wound Practice and Research. 2011;19(1):16–20.

Sillaber I, Henniger MS. Stress and alcohol drinking. Ann Med. 2004;36:596–605.

Silverstein P. Smoking and wound healing. Am J Med. 1992;93(1):B2–4.

Sinha R. Chronic stress, drug use, and vulnerability to addiction. Ann N Y Acad Sci. 2008;1141:105–30.

Solowiej K, Mason V, Upton D. Review of the relationship between stress and wound healing: part 1. J Wound Care. 2009;18(9):357–66.

Solowiej K, Mason V, Upton D. Psychological stress and pain in wound care, part 3: management. J Wound Care. 2010a;19(4):153–5.

Solowiej K, Mason V, Upton D. Psychological stress and pain in wound care, part 2: a review of pain and stress assessment tools. J Wound Care. 2010b;19(3):110–5.

Soon K, Acton C. Pain-induced stress: a barrier to wound healing. Wounds UK. 2006;2(4):92–101.

Spilsbury K, Nelson A, Cullum N, Iglesias C, Nixon J, Mason S. Pressure ulcers and their treatment and effects on quality of life: hospital inpatient perspectives. J Adv Nurs. 2007;57(5):494–504.

Taylor SE, Kemeny ME, Reed GM, Bower JE, Gruenewald TL. Psychological resources, positive illusions, and health. Am Psychol. 2000;55(1):99.

Thoits PA. Mechanisms linking social ties and support to physical and mental health. J Health Soc Behav. 2011;52(2):145–61.

Tønnesen H, Kehlet H. Preoperative alcoholism and postoperative morbidity. Br J Surg. 1999;86(7):869–74.

Trivedi RB, Bosworth HB, Jackson GL. Resilience in chronic illness. In: Resilience in aging. New York: Springer; 2011. p. 181–97.

Upton D. Psychological impact of pain in patients with wounds. London: Wounds UK; 2011a.

Upton D. Psychology of stress. In: Upton D, editor. Psychological impact of pain in patients with wounds. London: Wounds UK; 2011b.

Upton D, Andrews A. Negative pressure wound therapy: improving the patient experience, part two of three. J Wound Care. 2013a;22(11):582–91.

Upton D, Andrews A. Negative pressure wound therapy: improving the patient experience, part one of three. J Wound Care. 2013b; 22(10):552–7.

Upton D, Andrews A. Pain and trauma in negative pressure wound therapy: a review. Int Wound J. 2013c; Advance online publication.

Upton D, Hender C, Solowiej K. Mood disorders in patients with acute and chronic wounds: a health professional perspective. J Wound Care. 2012a;21(1):42–8.

Upton D, Hender C, Solowiej K, Woo K. Stress and pain associated with dressing change in chronic wound patients. J Wound Care. 2012b;22(2):53–61.

Upton D, Solowiej K, Hender C, Woodyat KY. Stress and pain associated with dressing change in patients with chronic wounds. J Wound Care. 2012c;21(2):53–61.

Upton D, Morgan J, Andrews A, et al. The pain and stress of wound treatment in patients with burns. An international burn specialist perspective. Wounds. 2013a;25(8):199–204.

Upton D, Stephens D, Andrews A. Patients' experience of negative pressure wound therapy. J Wound Care. 2013b;22(1):34–9.

Upton D, Thirlaway K. Promoting healthy lifestyles. 2nd ed. London: Routledge; 2014.

Van Loey NE, Van Son MJ. Psychopathology and psychological problems in patients with burn scars: epidemiology and management. Am J Clin Dermatol. 2003;4(4):245–72.

Vermeiden J, Doorn L, Da Costa A, Kaptein AA, Steenvoorde P. Coping strategies used by patients with chronic and/or complex wounds. Wounds. 2009;21(12):324–8.

Walshe C. Living with a venous leg ulcer: a descriptive study of patients' experiences. J Adv Nurs. 1995;22(6):1092–100.

Wilson RH, Wisely JA, Wearden AJ, Dunn KW, Edwards J, Tarrier N. Do illness perceptions and mood predict healing time for burn wounds? A prospective, preliminary study. J Psychosom Res. 2011;71(5):364–6. Epub 2011 Jul 12.

Woo KY. Wound-related pain: anxiety, stress and wound healing. Wounds UK. 2010;6(4):92–8.

Woo KY, Coutts PM, Price P, Harding K, Sibbald RG. A randomized crossover investigation of pain at dressing change comparing 2 foam dressings. Adv Skin Wound Care. 2009;22(7):304–10.

Chapter 2
Pain

> Box 2.1: Key Points
> - An understanding of pain and its impact on the individual is essential for wound care professionals;
> - The gate-control theory (GCT) of pain highlights that pain experience can be influenced by psychological, social and physiological factors;
> - Pain experienced during wound healing can negatively impact upon the patient experience, and ultimately, healing rate;
> - There is evidence supporting the link between psychosocial issues, stress, pain and delayed wound healing;
> - It is essential that clinicians assess all elements of pain in order to manage it appropriately and facilitate best wound care.

Summary

Pain is reported as being one of the most significant issues for the individual with a wound. Not only can it have a significant impact on quality of life, pain's intimate relationship with stress means that excessive pain can lead to stress and delayed healing. It is therefore essential that the health care professional understand how pain is best conceptualised, assessed and managed: this is the focus of this chapter. Detailing the pain associated with wounds precedes a description of the Gate Control Theory of Pain. This model highlights the importance of psychosocial variables in the experience of pain and how these components can also be used in the effective management of pain. In order to effectively manage pain it is necessary to assess pain appropriately and this chapter outlines several methods which can be used in wound care. Finally, approaches to pain management are presented.

Introduction

Pain and stress are two significant issues that can have a demonstrable impact not only on the patient experience but also on the healing of a patient's wound. As will be discussed, pain and stress are intrinsically linked and as such, pain has been found to have a major role in the patient's stress experience (Beitz and Goldberg 2005; Hareendran et al. 2005; Upton et al. 2012a, b, c). This can have significant consequences for wound care since increased levels of stress can lead to increased sensitivity to pain (Woo 2010). For example, it has been found that patients, who display significant levels of stress in anticipation of pain will, subsequently, rate their painful experience as more intense (Colloca and Benedetti 2007). Similarly, increased stress from the pain may lead to delayed healing (e.g. Upton et al. 2012a, b, c; see Chap. 3).

This and the subsequent chapter will explore these two fundamental issues, outline how they can be described and look at how wound healing is influenced by these related concepts. In this chapter, pain will be explored (see Box 2.1) before moving onto Chap. 3 which will explore stress and the inter-relationship between pain, stress and wound healing.

Research has highlighted the continual presence of pain associated with wounds, not only in relation to the wound itself but also during the wound-care regime (i.e. dressing change, wound manipulation, negative pressure treatment and so on) is significant- probably the most significant issue that those with wounds have to deal with. For example, it has been reported that 80 % of patients with venous leg ulcers report acute or chronic wound pain (Briggs and Nelson 2010). Additionally, half of these described their pain as moderate to the worst possible pain, a finding emphasised by patients' vivid memories and descriptions of such pain even after the wounds had healed. Research exploring pain in 32 patients with pressure ulcers echo such findings with 18 % reporting pain as excruciating or horrible, while 75 % highlighted the distress caused by such pain. Again, the distressing nature of wound pain has been elucidated by Price at al. (2008a, b), with patients perceiving such pain to be the most devastating aspect related to chronic wounds due to its all-encompassing nature.

Research has consistently highlighted the need for clinicians to incorporate both pain and stress management strategies into their care regimes. Despite this, however, health professionals often place lower importance on the management of pain, relegating it to a lower priority (Vermeulen et al. 2007). This is of substantial concern, particularly when (as will be discussed) the detrimental consequences associated with heightened pain are repeatedly reported. The vicious cycle of pain, stress, worsened pain and delayed wound healing has been evidenced substantially across wound related studies. As such, it is imperative that wound-care professionals are not only aware of this process, but also incorporate their knowledge and understanding of it within their clinical practice. The recognition of the primacy of pain and stress as part of the wound-care process and management can enhance not only wound healing, but also patients' overall psychological health and well-being.

Defining Pain

According to the International Association for the Study of Pain (IASP 2012), pain is defined as an unpleasant sensory and emotional experience associated with actual or potential tissue damage, or described in terms of such damage.

Pain is usually transitory, lasting only until the noxious stimulus is removed or the underlying damage or pathology has healed- this is acute pain. For example, acute pain may be exacerbated during regular treatment due to the need for manipulation; wound cleansing, dressing removal and re-application, debridement (White 2008; Upton 2011a, b).

However, some painful conditions may persist for years. This is chronic pain, as opposed to acute pain that may be experienced for a relatively brief period (e.g. during dressing change). The definition of chronic pain is rather arbitrary, however. The most commonly used definition being pain of greater than 3 or 6 months since the onset of pain (Turk and Okifuji 2002) though others have suggested a 12 month mark (Spanswick and Main 2000). Others apply *acute* to pain that lasts less than 30 days, *chronic* to pain of more than 6 months duration, and *subacute* to pain that lasts from 1 to 6 months (Thienhaus and Cole 2002). Alternatively, a compromise definition is that chronic pain is "pain that extends beyond the expected period of healing" (Turk and Okifuji 2002) and one that will be adopted here. Chronic pain may be an important component of care for patients with wounds given the potential chronicity of their wound and the regular requirement for dressing change.

In addition to the distinction between acute and chronic pain, there are many forms of pain, which may be useful to distinguish here. Hence, nociceptive pain is pain that happens because of tissue damage or inflammation and is caused by stimulation of peripheral nerve fibres that respond only to stimuli approaching or exceeding harmful intensity:

> Pain that arises from actual or threatened damage to non-neural tissue and is due to the activation of nociceptors (ISAP 2012)

Nociceptors are the nerves which sense and respond to parts of the body, which suffer from damage. They signal tissue irritation, impending injury, or actual injury. When activated, they transmit pain signals (via the peripheral nerves as well as the spinal cord) to the brain. This form of pain may be classified according to the mode of noxious stimulation (e.g. "thermal", "mechanical" or "chemical"). Examples include sprains, bone fractures, burns, bumps, bruises, inflammation (from an infection or arthritic disorder), obstructions, and myofascial pain (which may indicate abnormal muscle stresses). The pain is typically well localized, constant, and often with an aching or throbbing quality. Visceral pain is the subtype of nociceptive pain that involves the internal organs. It tends to be episodic and poorly localized.

In contrast, neuropathic pain is the pain associated with the nervous system and is the result of an injury or malfunction in the peripheral or central nervous system (Treede et al. 2008):

> Pain caused by a lesion or disease of the somatosensory nervous system (ISAP 2012)

Peripheral neuropathic pain is often described as "burning", "tingling", "electrical", "stabbing", or "pins and needles" (Paice 2003). Among the many causes of peripheral neuropathy, diabetes is the most common, but can also be caused by chronic alcohol use, exposure to other toxins (including many chemotherapies), vitamin deficiencies, and a large variety of other conditions. Persistent allodynia, pain resulting from a nonpainful stimulus such as a light touch, is also a common characteristic of neuropathic pain. The pain may persist for months or years beyond the apparent healing of any damaged tissues. In this setting, pain signals no longer represent an alarm about ongoing or impending injury, instead the alarm system itself is malfunctioning.

Finally, Phantom pain is pain felt in a part of the body that has been lost or from which the brain no longer receives signals. It is a type of neuropathic pain and is common in those with amputations (Kooijman et al. 2000).

It has been suggested that the pain that patients experience can be an issue for all irrespective of type of wound (see Table 2.1); whether chronic or acute (White 2008;

TABLE 2.1 Types of wound-related pain

Type	Cause	Duration
Chronic background pain	Neuropathic pain can occur from injury of trauma which causes nerve damage and subsequent malfunction of the central nervous system (CNS)	Neuropathic pain is often chronic and can last for months or years. The pain can become independent from the initial trauma or damage.
Pain at wound treatments	Nociceptive pain occurs when receptors (nociceptors) sense and respond to parts of the body that suffer from damage or trauma. It can be caused by trauma to a wound or the surrounding tissue when dressings are applied or removed. Wound cleansing (swabs, cold liquids, topical antiseptics) can also initiate acute pain.	Nociceptive pain can be both acute and persistent as a result of tissue damage. However, it is generally localised to the wound and the surrounding tissue.
Anticipatory pain	If patients perceive wound treatments to be painful from previous experience, this can initiate pain signals to the CNS. Patient anxiety can result in environmental and somatic signals being brought to the patient's attention, thus increasing sensory receptivity. Patients' expectations of pain at wound treatments can cause them to experience pain before the treatment has been administered.	Anticipatory pain is usually quite short in duration. It is dependent on the individual patient's perceptions.

Woo et al. 2008); or whether nocioceptive or neuropathic in origin (Soon and Acton 2006); or temporary or persistent. Krasner (1995) describes acute pain as cyclic (occurring during regular procedures) or non-cyclic (occurring during manipulation of wounds).

Furthermore since different forms of pain are often treated differently it is important for the health care professional to not only acknowledge any pain, but also correctly identify the type of pain in order to implement an accurate intervention. Finally, it should not be overlooked that wound pain is extremely distressing for patients and can result in the presentation of psychological problems, which can be costly both financially and emotionally for all (Upton and Hender 2012).

Patients have highlighted pain as being a significant stressor (Solowiej et al. 2009). This is particularly worrying when considering the body of research that has demonstrated the negative impact of stress in relation to wound healing (Cole-King et al. 2001; Soon and Acton 2006; Walburn et al. 2009). Hence, there is a need for clinicians and health professionals in the field of wound care to consider the assessment of wound pain, and any resultant stress, throughout the treatment process (see Chap. 3). Despite this, some health care providers have, traditionally, neglected pain and the need for its assessment and documentation (Woo et al. 2008). Indeed, many health-related organisations and care providers have highlighted the need for pain management to be incorporated into routine wound care practice. For example, the European Wound Management Association (EWMA) developed clinical guidelines and recommendations that highlighted best practice in relation to wound-pain assessment and management (European Wound Management Association 2002). Additionally, the World Union of Wound Healing Societies (WUWHS 2004) have emphasised the need for minimising wound-related pain. Within this consensus document, the WUWHS recommended the assessment of wound-related pain and its perceived intensity before, during and after dressing procedures. This is in the hope that, if needed, clinicians can review their practice if patients perceive their experience of pain to be of a rating of moderate or more (e.g. a pain score higher than 4 on a scale of 1–10). While clinicians have the tendency to consider would healing to be of utmost importance, patients consistently rate pain to be of most important to themselves.

In order to adequately treat pain, and attempt to negate its adverse effects, it is important to record when it occurs, while also identifying primary causes (White 2008). This would then enable the clinician to determine the most appropriate means for managing such pain including the application of supportive measures. There are a number of tools that can be adopted in assessing patient's pain throughout the treatment regime (some of which will be discussed later in this chapter). The adoption of these pain assessments would enable clinicians to alter regimes in an attempt to meet the needs of individual patients. Subsequently, the accurate assessment and management of wound pain can establish a basis of trust on the part of the patient, reduce the patient's overall pain and stress, contribute to patient quality of life (QoL) and increase treatment concordance (Hollinworth 2005; Upton and Solowiej 2010).

Models of Pain

There are, as one would expect, various models that have been developed in order to take into account the complex phenomena of pain and it is worth exploring some of these now in order to better understand the concept has been described, and subsequently how best to both assess and manage it (Upton 2012). Attempts at understanding pain have a long history, with one of the first explanations being provided by Descartes in 1644 who:

> Conceived of the pain system as a straight through channel from the skin to the brain (Melzack and Wall 1996:126).

In other words, when you hit your thumb with a hammer the hurt and damage from this area is sent up to the brain via one channel that tells you that you are experiencing pain.

This earlier view of pain as a simple linear concept was very popular up until the twentieth century when evidence to suggest that pain was not as simple as a mere linear relationship between injury and perceived pain started to mount up (Melzack and Wall 1996). Not only did evidence emerge that the level of pain was influenced by factors other than extent of injury- for example, personality, culture, anxiety and so on- but there was evidence that individuals with no nerve transmission could still experience pain. People who have lost limbs through amputation often have severe pain in the missing limbs. Thus, in those with phantom limb pain where there are no nerve transmissions but there is pain (e.g. Bosmans et al. 2010; Fieldsen and Wood 2011). Phantom limb pain has no physical basis but the pain can feel excruciating and feel as if it is spreading. Not only is the pain not related to actual tissue damage but not all people who have had a limb amputated experience this pain, or the level of pain may vary from individual to individual (Bosmans et al. 2010).

These pieces of evidence – the variation in medication's success at reducing pain, the variation in individual's perception of pain relating to the same tissue damage and pain without injury – indicate the pain process to be more complex than the linear-biomedical model, and that pain does not simply equate to injury. In response to this, the Gate Control Theory (GTC) was developed.

The Gate Control Theory (GTC) is probably the most influential theory of pain to date. This theory is said to have had a particularly important contribution to the understanding of pain due to the emphasis it places on the central neural mechanisms (Melzack 1999) and the appreciation that pain can be influenced by both a range of factors and not just those physiological ones related to the wound. Indeed, the gate-control theory was developed in order to account for the importance of both the mind and brain in the perception of pain (Melzack and Wall 1965). This particular theory, although accounting for primarily mental phenomena, considers the physiological basis in order to explain the complex phenomenon of pain. Thus, it established the brain as an active system that filters, selects and modulates inputs (Melzack 1999).

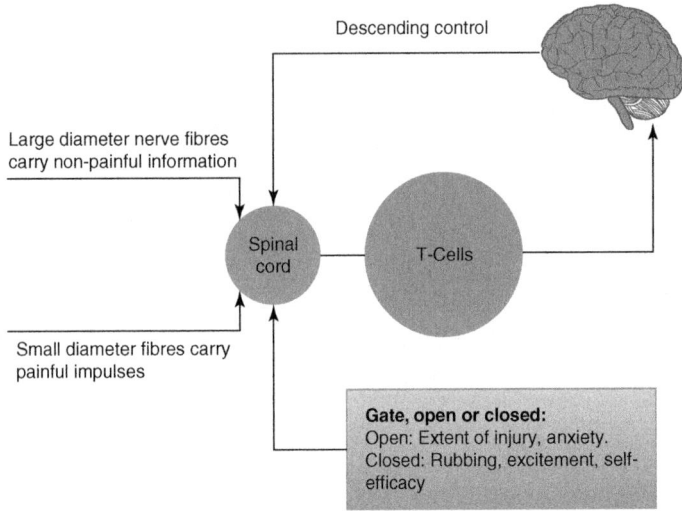

Figure 2.1 Gate control theory of pain (Adapted from Melzack and Wall (1965))

Specifically, it investigates the structure of the nervous system suggesting that the experience of pain is dependent on a complex interplay of these two systems; central nervous system and the peripheral nervous system.

Briefly, according to the GTC, when an injury occurs, pain messages originate within the nerves in the affected tissue and travel along the peripheral nerves to the spinal cord and then on up to the brain (see Fig. 2.1). However, before reaching the brain, the pain messages encounter a 'gate keeper' (a group of nerve cells known as the substantia gelatinosa situated within the spinal cord), which determines whether the pain signals proceed on to the brain or are blocked. This gate plays an important role in the pain management of the central nervous system. The substantia gelatinosa modulates sensory input through balancing the activity of small-diameter (*A-Delta and C*) and large-diameter (*A-beta*) fibres (Melzack 1996). Whilst large fibre activity (non-nociceptive) results in the closure of the spinal gating mechanism and prevention of synaptic transmission to centrally projecting T cells (transport cells),

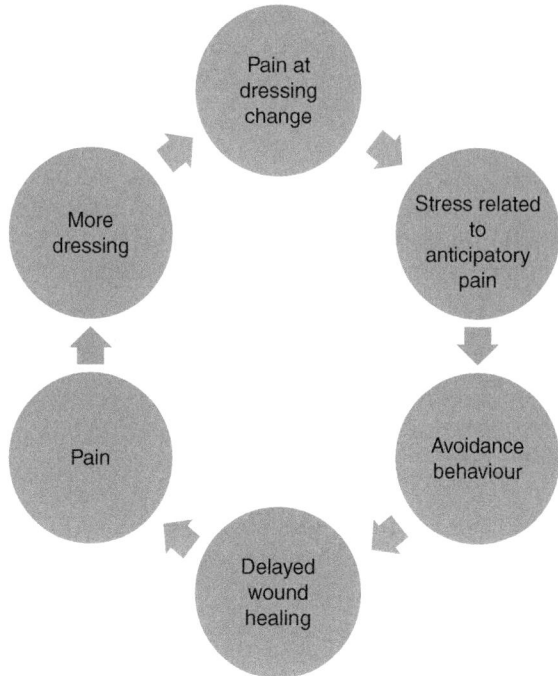

FIGURE 2.2 Cycle of pain, stress, wound healing and pain

activation of small fibres (nociceptive) open the gate and facilitate T cell activity (See Fig. 2.2). This activity is said to be responsible for the experience of pain (Weisenberg 1977).

Simply put, the GTC suggests that the pain messages on route to the brain are subject to a gate. If the gate is closed then less pain messages get through and, hence, less pain is experienced. In contrast, if the gate is open then potentially more pain is experienced. Both physiological (e.g. rubbing the wounded area) or psychological (e.g. stress or anxiety) can influence whether the gate is open or closed.

Within this theory, the experience of pain is seen as an on-going sequence of activities which is both reflexive and modifiable. The process described above results in overt communication and expressions of pain by the patients and the strategies they may adopt in order to control the painful experience. Furthermore, this theory allows for the management and shaping of painful experiences due to the multi-faceted nature of it (Novy et al. 1995). For example, in addition to the physiological aspects, it accounts for affective, behavioural, cognitive and sensory factors. Building upon the theory, Melzack (1993) argued that there was an interrelation of physiological and psychological facets, with affective, behavioural, cognitive and sensory-physical factors each being part of an integrated chronic pain system.

Although this theory has been subject to specific criticisms, particularly in relation to points of particular anatomical mechanisms, and suitably revised, it has been of enormous value in pushing forward and stimulating research surrounding the science of pain and the development of new clinical treatments (Melzack and Wall 1982). Furthermore, the model has led to the development of various pain management techniques, including that of neurophysiological procedures, behavioural treatments, pharmacological advance, and techniques targeted towards the alteration of attentional and perceptual pain associated processes (Novy et al. 1995).

Factors Influencing Pain

As discussed, pain is not a physiological symptom, but rather, a biopsychosocial phenomenon (Adams et al. 2006; Upton and Solowiej 2010). Pain, and its experience, is a complex and multi-faceted phenomenon, being subjective and often difficult to describe. In addition to the pathophysiological causes of wound pain, the patient's psychological state of mind, environment and cultural background can each impact on the way in which the patient perceives it (Briggs et al. 2002; Soon and Acton 2006; see Table 2.2). Indeed, there are whole ranges of factors that can influence whether the gate is open or closed, for example:

- The amount of activity in the pain fibres: the greater the injury the more active the pain fibres, the more open the gate, meaning larger injuries often cause more pain than smaller ones.

TABLE 2.2 Factors influencing pain

	Opens the gate	**Closes the gate**
Emotional factors	Anxiety	Happiness
	Worry	Optimism
	Tension	Relaxation
	Depression	
Cognitive and behavioural factors	Focusing on the pain	More involvement and interest in life activities
	Boredom	Distractions or focus on other activities
	Other reactions	Other reactions
Physical factors	Extent and type of injury	Medication
	Low activity level	Counter-stimulation (e.g. rubbing)

- The amount of activity in other peripheral fibres: some small fibres and A-beta fibres, carry information about harmless stimuli (e.g. touching or rubbing of the skin) and tend to close the gate. This is why you can rub a cut better.
- Messages that descend from the brain: impulses from neurons in the brainstem and cortex can open or close the gate. The effects of some of these (e.g. anxiety or excitement) may open or close the gate, so what would normally bring a child to tears goes unnoticed when they are having fun with their friends at their birthday party. Similarly, self-efficacy – the extent to which somebody believes they are able to cope with pain – can influence their pain perception (Walker 2001). Research has also shown that anxiety can lead to increased self reported pain intensity (Jones et al. 2002), reduced pain tolerance (Carter et al. 2002), and decreased pressure pain thresholds (Michelotti et al. 2000).

Pathophysiological causes of pain can include wound aetiology, pressure from neoplasms, prolonged inflammation, hypersensitivities, venous insufficiency and vacuities, or even local infection (Hollinworth 2005). Additionally, pain can be exacerbated through psychological causes. For example, the experience of pain can cause a patient to experience an abundance of negative emotional states including those of fear, anxiety and depression (Woo et al. 2008). Through a complex interaction, such negative states can lead to psychological stress and the reduction of a patient's pain threshold and subsequent pain tolerance (Woo et al. 2008). This results in a continuous cycle of increased pain – stress – and subsequent pain, negatively impacting upon wound healing.

Psychological Influences, Pain and Stress

It has been found that the chronic pain, as highlighted above, can lead to inadequate adaption to living with a wound, negatively impacting upon a patient's psychological functioning (Upton 2011a, b). Extreme or exaggerated wound pain can lead to patient's experiencing higher forms of distress, frustrations and lowered self-esteem. In addition to this, patients can experience severe emotional and physical stress (see Chap. 3). Such psychological factors (stress in particular) can have a significant impact on the way that a patient perceives their experience of pain. This emotional response can affect both biological and behavioural responses, subsequently impacting, again, on the emotional response to pain, resulting in a continuous negative cycle.

There is a recurring theme with regards to a patient's experience of pain: stress and subsequent further pain. The initial pain that patients experience due to their wound can lead to heightened levels of stress and anxiety. In turn, this stress lowers the patient's tolerance and pain threshold, subsequently resulting in the experience of worsened pain (Woo 2010).

Assessing Pain

Due to the negative impact of pain (and stress) on the rate of a patient's healing process and quality of life, assessing and measuring this is fundamental during the wound care process. It is essential that pain is assessed, managed and re-assessed regularly during a patient's treatment (Soon and Acton 2006). The need for consideration of pain on an individual patient basis has been highlighted by the World Union of Wound Healing Societies:

> Every person and every wound should have an individualised management plan: uncontrolled pain should signal an immediate adjustment to the plan. Wounds differ in their origins and prospects of healing, which has potential implications for the likelihood and severity of pain experienced, and should guide the choice of treatment options and strategies used in dressing related procedures. The aims is to treat all causes of pain and the clinicians will need to consider the patient's level of background and incident pain prior to any clinical intervention. (WUWHS 2004)

In implementing some form of assessment tool developed to measure pain, a clinician is aware of both the pain and stress experienced by their patient, enabling them to focus more specifically on contributing factors. This, subsequently, can aid the patient's rate of healing. As such, a patient-centred assessment can provide the clinician with a sensitive and effective tool for the management of wound-related pain (Upton and Solowiej 2010). Not only is it important for clinicians to adopt formal assessments, but it is also important for them to acknowledge individual patient behaviours; both verbal and non-verbal (see Table 2.3 for a non-verbal checklist). These behaviours can be indicative of instances of pain, whilst also enabling professionals to understand the varying levels of pain patients are experiencing during their woundcare (Upton and Solowiej 2010).

Clinicians have a number of self-report pain measures that they can adopt in their wound care and treatment regime (some, of which, will be outlined below). These measures

Table 2.3 Checklist of non-verbal pain indicators

Vocal Expressions	Moans, grunts, cries, sighs, gasps.
Facial Expressions	Winces, grimace, furrowed brow, tightened lips, jaw drop, clench teeth.
Bracing	Clutching/holding bed rails, tray or table, or affected area of pain.
Restlessness	Shifting position, hand movements, unable to keep still.
Rubbing	Touching, holding, rubbing or massaging affected area.

Adapted from Feldt (2000)

often adopt a scale or index format in order to determine the amount of pain patients are experiencing during their wound-related care. Measures of pain often include an index or scale to determine the amount of pain experienced by the patient. This is demonstrated in a number of ways amongst the measures shown in Table 2.4.

Verbal Pain Rating Scale (VPRS)/Numerical Pain Rating Scale (NPRS)

These self-report scales can be administered to patients and require them to define their pain from a list of descriptive words such as mild, discomforting or excruciating (i.e. a Verbal Pain Rating Scale- VPRS), or numerically, such as, 0 = no pain to, 100 = severe pain (i.e. a Numerical Pain Rating Scale- NPRS). Both these types of scales can be advantageous for the health professional in that they can be administered to measure pain intensity at differing intervals, over a period of time in a simple and efficient manner. They are easy to understand by both the patient and the clinician. However, such scales may be inaccurate due to the potential for patients to recall previous ratings, thus influencing their current rating.

TABLE 2.4 An evaluation of a selection of self-report methods designed to measure pain

Measure	Purpose	Strengths	Weaknesses
McGill Pain Questionnaire (MPQ), (Melzack 1975)	Assesses the different components of reported pain, how pain changes over time, and what things relieve or increase it. Also includes a measure of pain intensity.	Widely used, well-known pain report measure. Provides quantitative information that can be treated statistically, and is sufficiently sensitive to detect differences among different methods to relieve pain.	Long and potentially time consuming
Verbal Pain Rating Scale (VPRS)	The scale consists of a list of words describing different levels of pain; patients indicate their current level of pain by ticking the box next to the appropriate word. Descriptors are given a score (least painful = 0, most painful = 5), higher scores reflect more intense pain.	Easy to administer. Can be used to measure pain at intervals, over time.	When taking a series of measurements over time, patients may be able to recall their previous scores, thus not producing a true reflection of their reported pain.

(continued)

Chapter 2. Pain

TABLE 2.4 (continued)

Measure	Purpose	Strengths	Weaknesses
Numerical Pain Rating Scale (NPRS)	The scale requires the patient to define the intensity of their pain in numerical terms between 0 (no pain) – 100 (severe pain) by writing their number of choice on the scale. Higher scores indicate more severe pain.	Easy to administer. Can be used to measure pain at intervals, over time.	When taking a series of measurements over time, patients may be able to recall their previous scores, thus not producing a true reflection of their reported pain.
Wong Faces Scale	Patient rates the intensity of the pain on a six point scale, with the higher the score the greater the pain. Pain ratings are represented by faces illustrating greater pain.	Easy to administer and can be used with those with low verbal skills.	Some questions over the validity of the questionnaire in elderly patients or those with a cognitive impairment.

Visual Analogue Scale (VAS)

This self-reported measure entails drawing a cross or mark somewhere on a pre-defined line (usually 10 cm in length) with pain descriptors on either end, enabling the clinician to determine their patient's pain intensity. This, more abstract, measure reduces the ability for patient's to recall where they previously located their pain. Subsequently, the effects of practice bias that may be evident with the VPRS and NPRS are significantly reduced.

The McGill Pain Questionnaire (MPQ; Melzack and Wall 1996)

Another more multi-faceted assessment tool is the MPQ. This measure is designed to account for various components, including the description and location of pain, changes in pain over time and factors that relieve or increase pain. This is in conjunction with a measure of pain intensity. A significant advantage if the MPQ is its ability and sensitivity to changes in treatment regime, enabling clinicians to assess and compare patient's experiences of pain over a length of time. In addition to this, the MPQ can provide clinicians with detailed information of particular treatment strategies in relation to multiple dimensions of pain (sensory, affective and evaluative).

The Faces Pain Scale (Hockenberry et al. 2005)

The Faces Pain Scale is a simple six point scale that was initially developed for children but has subsequently been used in those with a cognitive impairment or the elderly.

Although the Faces Pain Scale is extensively used and simple to implement, it has been noted that there were "raising serious doubts about the validity of the Faces Pain Scale as a measure of pain in older adults. This problem is even more marked when nursing home residents and older adults with mild cognitive impairment are asked to put the faces in the correct order. The Faces Pain Scale cannot, therefore, be recommended for general clinical use with older adults or nursing home residents" (British Pain Society and British Geriatrics Society 2007).

Pain Management

If we consider the links that have been established between the experience of wound-related pain and the occurrence of psychological distress, it could be argued that if wound-pain were to be managed accurately, psychological stress may reduce substantially and their quality of life would increase. That is, if the pain a patient experiences at dressing change or wound manipulation is managed and subsequently reduced, the pain-stress-pain cycle highlighted above may be interrupted, consequently resulting in improved wound healing and psychological health. So, how can pain be best managed?

One particular model that can prove effective in appropriately managing a patient's wound-related pain is the P.A.I.N. model developed by Keyte and Richardson (2011). This model consists of four elements, Preparation, Assessment, Intervention and Normalisation, each of which will be briefly outlined below.

Preparation

In order to appropriately manage pain it is essential to acknowledge it as a biopsychosocial phenomenon. Thus, it is necessary to consider not only the physiology but also the social contexts and psychological aspects of pain. In order to facilitate pain and stress management appropriately it is imperative that, within the preparation stage, excellent interpersonal skills and a good therapeutic relationship is established. Care regimes need to include environmental strategies that create a relaxed situation where patients feel

Table 2.5 Pain variations in acute and chronic pain

Wound Type	Pain Type
Acute	Acute background pain
Acute	Acute/procedural pain during dressing change
Chronic	Chronic nociceptive background pain
Chronic	Chronic neuropathic background pain
Chronic	Acute/procedural pain during dressing change
Chronic	Neuropathic pain during dressing change

comfortable and practitioners are able to reach optimal pain management. As neuropathic pains may present unusual symptoms (such as allodynia or hyperalgesia), clinicians may encounter novel situations whereby patient's experiences of pain vary despite similarities in the presentation of their wounds. Hence, within the preparation stage, it is necessary for clinicians to consider their own thoughts and feelings in relation to wound treatment and pain to encourage open-mindedness and non-pejorative approaches. Additionally, it is essential that clinicians recognise that acute pain and chronic pain require different skills in terms of management (IASP 2012).

Assessment

Next, in providing effective pain management, clinicians need to accurately assess patient's experiences of pain (as described above). This can sometimes be troublesome due to the complex nature of wound treatment (various forms of wounds and pain see Table 2.5), requiring clinicians to compartmentalise the numerous aspects of pain and wound care. Hence, an individualised approach is needed with practitioners adopting a flexible and open-minded attitude to differing treatment regimes.

In assessing acute and procedural pain, clinicians can adopt a variety of measures, including those outlined above. Although these assessments can provide clinicians with an insight into their patient's experience of pain, it is necessary to combine these scores with anecdotal experience in order to identify potential magnification or underplaying of pain intensity. As such, an individualised, patient-centred approach is essential (Nielsen et al. 2009). Chronic pain, however, differs in that patients experiencing this type of pain can show little variation in its intensity over time (Stomski et al. 2010). Hence, intensity score such as the VAS may prove ineffective. Rather, it is more appropriate to use measures such as the MPQ. In doing so, the clinician can gain a deeper understanding of the contributing factors of increased and reduced pain. Taking the time to consider patient's experience of pain, and on pain experienced during previous treatment and dressing regimes, can equip clinicians with the understanding and knowledge of how to accurately manage that pain. Thus, multi-dimensional measures such as that of the MPQ can account for all the biopsychosocial elements needed in doing this.

Intervention

A multi-modal approach to pain management is more effective than a single pharmacological agent (Hollinworth 2005; White 2008). Not only does this approach need to be implemented when managing on-going wound pain, but is also important when approaching the problematic pain inducing nature of dressing change (Upton 2011a, b; Woo et al. 2009). The multi-modal approach to pain management is one which is embedded within the World Health Organisation (WHO) analgesic ladder (WHO 2010) into practice. It is particularly effective in relation to pain management in that it ensures that all pain pathways are targeted in an attempt to relieve patients' experience of pain.

There are a number of analgesic medications which can prove useful in targeting pain, differing in relation to wound and pain type. Firstly, bottom of the WHO ladder, paracetamol is a widespread analgesic which should be used as a basis for management of both acute and chronic pain and wounds, being used continuously with consistent chronic pain or 1 h before a dressing change (if pain is only experienced during dressing change). Additionally, non-steroidal anti-inflammatory drugs (NSAIDs) have an analgesic and anti-inflammatory effect, reducing the sensitisation to pain. They can be used in conjunction with paracetamol as no compatibility issues have been discovered and, again, can be used to treat both continuous background and dressing procedural-related pain for all types of wounds. However, NSAIDs have been found to have side-effects including gastric irritation and the potential for cardiac and renal compromise (Upton 2011a, b).

Next on the WHO ladder is the addition of weak opioids such as codeine. If a combination of paracetamol and NSAIDs are not sufficient in managing background wound pain, the addition of a weak opioid at a dosing frequency relative to the management of pain should be administered. However, codeine can have variable efficacy due to it being a pro-drug requiring modification into an active drug before effect using the enzyme CYP2D6 (Stamer and Stuber 2007). This particular enzyme, however, is not active, or is significantly lower, in some patients proving ineffective in approximately 10 % of the population or even as high as 40 % with highly stressed populations (Poulsen et al. 1998). Hence, if on repeat doses clinicians become aware of non-deliverance of analgesia, alternative weak opioids such as tramadol need to be administered.

Finally, at the top of the WHO analgesic ladder is the strong opioid, Morphine, and is only administered if pain has not be adequately relieved via the combined analgesia suggested by the previous WHO steps. Morphine can be administered via all routes being flexibly dosed at a quantity suitable for individual patients. However, only on rare occasions should morphine be administered for wound-related background pain. Clinicians need to be aware of patient's healing progress in order to reduce its dosage as soon as the pain lessens. It can also be used for dressing change-related pain but, as with the previous analgesics, it should be delivered an hour before treatment. Additionally, clinicians need to be aware of the actions and side-effects of opioids in order to achieve good analgesia appropriate for pain management. Side-effects may include constipation, nausea/vomiting, sedation and respiratory depression (McNicol et al. 2003). When used solely for dressing change, practitioners need to observe for each of these side-effects at each dose administration. Pain can act as an antidote to respiratory depression although, if administered during preparation for dressing change (hence, a currently pain-free period), it is essential to monitor the patients and their safety.

In addition to the analgesics within the WHO ladder, there are co-analgesics that treat non-nociceptive elements of pain. Although neuropathic pain and its associated symptoms (including allodynia and hyperalgesia) are coincident with nociceptive pain, they are unresponsive to the same drugs used in the management of nociceptive pain. Differing to nociceptive pain, neuropathic pain stems from within the nerves themselves, thus medication targeting this area is essential. Antidepressive and anticonvulsant co-analgesics such as amitriptyline and gabapentin have proven useful in managing such pain. However, clinicians should begin with low doses, increasing if need be whilst accounting for potential side-effects.

Other pain management strategies can implement the use of nitrous oxide, most commonly the 50:50 strength mixture with that of oxygen. Although its mode of action for analgesia is unclear, it is often useful when managing painful dressing changes. It has very few side-effects and can be self-administered via a mouthpiece or facemask. Thus, the patient can inhale the substance in accordance with their perceived pain. Additionally, nitrous oxide can be used in addition to other analgesics with no contraindications. There are limited disadvantages to the use of nitrous oxide and numerous advantages. Firstly, training in the administration of the equipment is relatively simple and quick, the equipment is portable, and most forms of the 50:50 mixture are relatively cheap to buy. Despite this, some health providers have highlighted concerns over the repeated exposure to nitrous oxide, although the majority of wound care clinicians would be significantly below the limits proposed by the Health and Safety Committee in relation to its use.

Limited evidence is available in relation to the effectiveness of complementary therapies in the management of wounds and wound-related pain. That said it would be inaccurate to suggest that complementary therapies do not work. Conversely, as suggested in the preparation element of the P.A.I.N model, in order to maximise the efficacy of management techniques, it is essential to control the psychological state of the patient. Hence, the relaxation component included in complementary therapies is highly advantageous to the pain-management process. There are a number of non-pharmacological interventions considered useful for the care and management of wound, although the coverage of these is beyond the remit of this book. Nonetheless, recent publications have discussed one specific non-pharmacological issue associated with wound care.

In a review of the psychological models that have been used to conceptualise chronic pain, Turk et al. (2008) suggested that a more realistic approach to eliminate pain will likely combine pharmacological, physical and psychological components tailored to each patient's needs. In their review, the greatest empirical evidence for success with psychological interventions was found for Cognitive-Behavioural Therapy (CBT) which includes stress management, problem solving, meditation, relaxation and goal setting. In CBT, therapists help patients build their communication skills, gain a sense of control over their pain and cope with the fear of pain. Patients are taught positive coping strategies so that they will gain control over their pain, resulting in improved mood (Turk et al. 2008).

It has been discovered that when dressings are applied to a patient's wound it can create analgesia (Charles et al. 2002; MacBride et al. 2008), although it is not clear whether this is, in part, due to the extreme pain experienced during the dressing

TABLE 2.6 Potential mechanisms of analgesic properties of dressings (Richardson and Upton 2010)

Out of sight, out of mind
The dressing as a protector
Moist environment – bathing of nociceptors
Moist environment – control of inflammation and hyperalgesia
Moist environment – recruitment of analgesic compounds to the wound area
Temperature change – generating heat or cooling effects
Counter-irritation
Removal of irritant exudate
The sequestration of pro-inflammatory cytokines
The direct influence of the dressing material

change procedure. When considering the pathways initiated during the experience of painful sensations, ten mechanisms have been identified for the analgesic properties of dressings (Richardson and Upton 2010; Table 2.6). The identification of such mechanisms is needed in order to, subsequently, test them. Psychological factors are an essential component of these mechanisms, which leads us to the final stage of the P.A.I.N. model of pain management, normalisation.

Normalisation

This final stage of the pain management model aims to return the patient to their original or new optimal condition, resulting in little or no painful effect on on-going activities. Anticipation of pain has been found to activate similar areas of the brain to that of actual pain (Fairhurst et al. 2007; Watson et al. 2009). Consequently, it is essential that the clinician use normalisation techniques in order to counter the anticipation, resulting in a pain-free dressing change and lowered anxiety. In controlling anxiety, it patients with prolonged experience of painful dressing change may need more than a single-pain free experiences. Sometimes, in such situations, the clinician may need to implement a separate strategy for the management of patient anxiety.

Summary

Pain is a complex phenomenon with a multitude of influential factors, including social, psychological and physiological elements. It is important for clinicians to consider these multiple factors and the techniques available to them when dealing with wounds. The reduction of pain can have a significant positive impact upon both the physical health and psychological health of a patient. Hence, it is essential that clinicians acknowledge, assess, and manage the presence of pain appropriately and effectively. In implementing such strategies it is suggested that the pain-stress-pain cycle can be broken, enabling the facilitation of wound healing whilst also improving patient's experience of wound management, health and subsequent quality of life.

References

Adams N, Poole H, Richardson C. Psychological approaches to chronic pain management. J Clin Nurs. 2006;15:290–300.
Beitz JM, Goldberg E. The lived experience of having a chronic wound: a phenomenologic study. J Medsurg Nurs. 2005;14(1):51–62.
Bosmans JC, Geertzen JHB, Post W, Van der Schans CP, Dijkstra PU. Factors associated with phantom limb pain: a 3 ½ year prospective study. Clin Rehabil. 2010;24(5):444–53.
Briggs M, Nelson EA. Topical agents or dressings for pain in venous leg ulcers. Cochrane Database Syst Rev. 2010;4:1–32.
Briggs M, Torra I, Bou JE. Pain at wound dressing changes: a guide to management. European Wound Management Association position document. London: Medical Education Partnership Ltd; 2002. p. 12–7.
British Pain Society and British Geriatrics Society. Guidance on the assessment of pain in older people. 2007. Available from:

http://www.gloucestershire.gov.uk/extra/CHttpHandler.ashx?id=45208&p=0.

Carter LE, McNeil DW, Vowles KE, Sorrell JT, Turk CL, Ries BJ, Hopko DR. Effects of emotion of pain reports, tolerance and physiology. Pain Res Manag. 2002;7:21–30.

Charles H, Callicot C, Mathurin D, Ballard K, Hart J. Randomised, comparative study of three primary dressings for the treatment of venous ulcers. Br J Community Nurs. 2002;7(6):48–54.

Cole-King A, Harding KG. Psychological factors and delayed healing in chronic wounds. Psychosom Med. 2001;63:216–20.

Colloca L, Benedetti F. Nocebo Hyperalgesia: how anxiety is turned into pain. Curr Opin Anaesthesiol. 2007;20(5):435–9.

European Wound Management Association. Pain at dressing changes. EWMA position document. London: MEP Ltd; 2002.

Fairhurst M, Wiech K, Dunckley P, Tracey I. Anticipatory brainstem activity predicts neural processing of pain in humans. Pain. 2007;128:101–10.

Feldt K. The checklist of non-vergal pain indicators (CNPL). Pain Manag Nurs. 2000;1(1):13–21.

Fieldsen D, Wood S. Dealing with phantom limb pain after amputation. Nurs Times. 2011;107(1):21–3.

Hareendran A, Bradbury A, Budd J, Geroulakos G, Hobbs R, Kenkre J, Symonds T. Measuring the impact of venous leg ulcers on quality of life. J Wound Care. 2005;14(2):53–7.

Hockenberry M, Wilson D, Winkelstein M. Wong's essentials of paediatric nursing. 7th ed. St. Louis: Mosby; 2005.

Hollinworth H. The management of patients' pain in wound care. Nurs Stand. 2005;20(7):65–73.

IASP. International Association for the Study of pain taxonomy. 2012. Available from: http://www.iasp-pain.org/Education/Content.aspx?ItemNumber=1698.

Jones A, Spindler H, Jorgensen MM, Zachariae R. The effect of situation-evoked anxiety and gender on pain report using the cold pressor test. Scand J Psychol. 2002;43(4):307–13.

Keyte D, Richardson C. Re-thinking pain educational strategies: pain a new model using e-learning and PBL. Nurse Educ Today. 2011;31(2):117–21.

Kooijman CM, Dijkstra PU, Geertzen JHB, Elzinga A, van der Schans CP. Phantom pain and phantom sensations in upper limb amputees: an epidemiological study. Pain. 2000;87(1):33–41.

Krasner D. The chronic wound pain experience: a conceptual model. Ostomy Wound Manage. 1995;41(3):20–5.

MacBride S, Wells ME, Hornsby C, Sharp L, Finnila K, Downie L. A case study to evaluate a new soft silicone dressing, Mepilex lite, for patients with radiation skin reactions. Cancer Nurs. 2008;31(1):8–14.

McNicol E, Horowicz-Mehler N, Fisk RA. Management of opioid side effects in cancer-related and chronic non-cancer pain. A systematic review. J Pain. 2003;4(4):231–56.

Melzack R. The McGill pain questionnaire: major properties and scoring methods. J Pain. 1975;1(3):277–99.

Melzack R. Pain: past present and future. Can J Exp Psychol. 1993;47: 615–29.

Melzack R. Gate control theory: on the evolution of pain concepts. J Pain. 1996;5:128–38.

Melzack R. From the gate to the neuromatrix. Pain. 1999;82(1):121–6.

Melzack R, Wall PD. Pain mechanisms: a new theory. Science. 1965;150:971–9.

Melzack R, Wall P. The challenge of pain. London: Penguin; 1982.

Melzack R, Wall PD. The challenge of pain. 2nd ed. New York: Penguin Books; 1996.

Michelotti A, Farella M, Tedesco A, Cimino R, Martina R. Changes in pressure-pain thresholds of the jaw muscles during a natural stressful condition in a group of symptom-free subjects. J Orafac Pain. 2000;14(4):279–85.

Nielsen CS, Staud R, Price DD. Individual differences in pain sensitivity: measurement, causation, and consequences. J Pain. 2009; 10(3):231–7.

Novy MD, Nelson VD, Francis JD, Turk CD. Perspectives of chronic pain: an evaluative comparison of restrictive and comprehensive models. Psychol Bull. 1995;118(2):238–47.

Paice JA. Mechanisms and management of neuropathic pain in cancer. J Support Oncol. 2003;1(2):107–20.

Poulsen L, Riishede L, Brosen K, Clemensen S, Sindrup SH. Codeine in post-operative pain: study of the influence of sparteine phenotype and serum concentrations of morphine and morphine-6-glucoronide. Eur J Clin Pharmacol. 1998;54(4):451–4.

Price JR, Mitchell E, Tidy E, Hunot V. Cognitive behaviour therapy for chronic fatigue syndrome in adults. Cochrane Database Syst Rev. 2008;(3):CD0010207

Price PE, Fagervik-Morton H, Mudge EJ, Beele H, Conteras Ruiz J, Huldt Nystrom T, Harding KG. Dressing- related pain in patients with chronic wounds: an international patient perspective. Int Wound J. 2008b;5(2):159–71.

Richardson C, Upton D. A discussion of the potential mechanisms for wound dressings' apparent analgesic effects. J Wound Care. 2010;19(10):424–30.

Solowiej K, Mason V, Upton D. Review of the relationship between stress and wound healing: part 1. J Wound Care. 2009;18(9): 357–66.

Soon K, Acton C. Pain-induced stress: a barrier to wound healing. Wounds UK. 2006;2(4):92–101.

Spanswick CC, Main CJ. Pain management: an interdisciplinary approach. Edinburgh: Churchill Livingstone; 2000.

Stamer UM, Stuber F. Genetic factors in pain and its treatment. Curr Opin Anaesthesiol. 2007;20(5):478–84.

Stomski NJ, Mackintosh S, Stanley M. Patient self-report measures of chronic pain consultation measures: a systematic review. Clin J Pain. 2010;26(3):235–43.

Thienhaus O, Cole BE. Classification of pain. In: Weiner R, editor. Pain management: a practical guide for clinicians. Boca Raton: CRC Press; 2002.

Treede RD, Jensen TS, Campbell JN, Cruccu G, Dostrovsky JO, Griffin JW, et al. Neuropathic pain: redefinition and a grading system for clinical and research purposes. Neurology. 2008;70(18):1630–5.

Turk DC, Okifuji A. Psychological factors in chronic pain: evolution and revolution. J Consult Clin Psychol. 2002;70(3):678–90.

Turk DC, Swanson KS, Tunks ER. Psychological approaches in the treatment of chronic pain patients: when pills, scalpels and needles are not enough. Can J Psychiatry. 2008;53(4):213–23.

Upton D. Psychological impact of pain in patients with wounds. London: Wounds UK; 2011a.

Upton D. Psychology of stress. In: Upton D, editor. Psychological impact of pain in patients with wounds. London: Wounds UK; 2011b.

Upton D. Introducing psychology for nurses and healthcare professionals. Edinburgh: Pearson; 2012.

Upton D, Hender C. The cost of mood disorder in patients with chronic wounds. Wounds UK. 2012;8(1):107–9.

Upton D, Solowiej K. Pain and stress as contributors to delayed wound healing. Wound Pract Res. 2010;18(3):114–22.

Upton D, Hender C, Solowiej K. Mood disorders in patients with acute and chronic wounds: a health professional perspective. J Wound Care. 2012a;21(1):42–8.

Upton D, Hender C, Solowiej K, Woo K. Stress and pain associated with dressing change in chronic wound patients. J Wound Care. 2012b;22(2):53–61.

Upton D, Solowiej K, Hender C, Woodyat KY. Stress and pain associated with dressing change in patients with chronic wounds. J Wound Care. 2012c;21(2):53–61.

Vermeulen H, van Hattem JM, Storm-Versloot MN, Ubbink DT, Westerbos SJ. Topical silver for treating infected wounds. Cochrane Database Syst Rev 2007;(1):4–27.

Walburn J, Vedhara K, Hankins M, Rixon L, Weinman J. Psychological stress and wound healing in humans: a systematic review and meta-analysis. J Psychosom Res. 2009;67:253–71.

Walker J. Control and the psychology of health. Buckingham: Open University Press; 2001.

Watson A, El-Deredy W, Domenico Iannetti G. Placebo conditioning and placebo analgesia modulate a common brain network during pain anticipation and perception. J Pain. 2009;145:24–30.

Weisenberg M. Pain and pain control. Psychol Bull. 1977;84:1008–44.

White R. A multinational survey of the assessment of pain when removing dressings. Wounds UK. 2008;4(1):1–6.

Woo KY. Wound-related pain: anxiety, stress and wound healing. Wounds UK. 2010;6(4):92–8.

Woo KY, Harding K, Price P, Sibbald G. Minimising wound-related pain at dressing change: evidence-informed practice. Int Wound J. 2008;5(2):144–57.

Woo KY, Coutts PM, Price P, Harding K, Sibbald RG. A randomized crossover investigation of pain at dressing change comparing 2 foam dressings. Adv Skin Wound Care. 2009;22(7):304–10.

World Health Organization. The pain analgesic ladder. WHO, Geneva. 2010. Available online at: www.who.int/cancer/palliative/painladder/en.

World Union of Wound Healing Societies. Principles of best practise: minimising pain at wound dressing-related procedures: a consensus document. London: MEP; 2004.

Chapter 3
Stress

> Box 3.1: Key Points
> - Stress can have a significant impact on wound healing;
> - Stress can be a consequence of the wound, social isolation, psychological issues, pain from the wound and pain from the treatment regimen;
> - The interactional model of stress suggests stress is a transaction between an individual and their environment – an event only elicits a stress response if the individual perceives the event to be stressful;
> - The General Adaptation Syndrome (GAS) describes three stages associated with stress: alarm, resistance, and exhaustion stage;
> - The importance of perception in the understanding of stress and how this can be applied to wound treatment is emphasised.

Summary

The relationship between stress and delayed healing is now firmly established. This evidenced relationship may be associated with a range of factors linked to wound care.

For example, the novelty of certain treatments- negative pressure for example- or the pain associated with wound management. Given the range of factors that are associated with wound related stress it is important that the health care professional understands the nature and model of stress, how best to assess it in practice and how any stress can be managed. These will be the foci of this particular chapter. Stress may be a consequence of several wound related factors: most particularly pain and wound management pain in particular. Preventing stress, and stress related to pain, is important not just for the relationship with delayed wound healing, but importantly, to understand that this may be an ongoing deleterious cyclical relationship. Increased wound related pain leads to increased stress which leads to delayed healing, which can lead to more pain. It is this cycle that this chapter addresses and suggests methods to break this damaging predicament.

Introduction

Many clinicians, when asked, believe that there is a relationship between stress and delayed healing (Upton and Solowiej 2011). It is evident from the research literature that there is strong empirical support for this belief (Broadbent et al. 2003; Ebrecht et al. 2004; Francis and Pennebaker 1992; Gouin et al. 2008; Jones et al. 2006; Marucha et al. 1998; Weinman et al. 2008; Kiecolt-Glaser et al. 1995; Glaser et al. 1999; Cole-King and Harding 2001) with a major theme suggesting that interventions need to be implemented as part of the wound care process in order to minimise patients' psychological stress/anxiety. This delayed healing may be evident in both acute and chronic wounds. For example, wound healing is a critical outcome in acute surgical wounds (Broadbent et al. 2003). Poor healing can result in wound infections or complications, as well as prolonged hospital stays, increased patient discomfort, and delayed return to activity (Broadbent et al. 2003). It is therefore important to maximise the healing rate by minimising any stress (see Box 3.1).

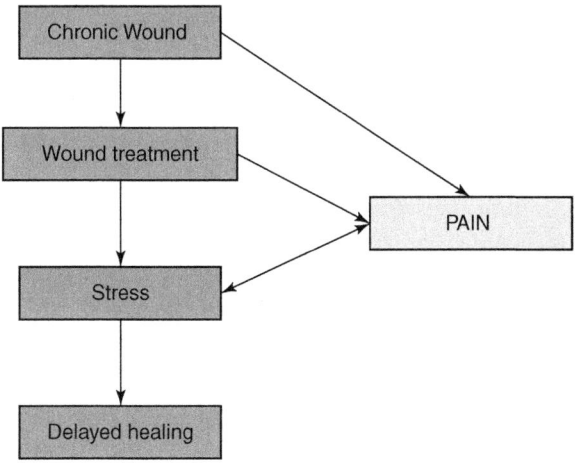

FIGURE 3.1 A model illustrating link between psychological stress, pain and chronic wound healing

In the Broadbent et al. study (2003), a sample of 47 patients with an inguinal hernia were given a standardised questionnaire assessing psychological stress and worry about the operation before undergoing open incision repair. Greater worry about the operation predicted more painful, poorer and slower recovery. These results also suggest that in clinical practice, interventions to reduce the patient's psychological stress may improve wound repair and healing, and facilitate recovery following surgery.

A similar pattern, albeit for different reasons, exists with chronic wounds. Psychological stress can be experienced in the presence of pain in chronic wounds so that the pain itself is seen as a stressor. Stress can also be induced by the anticipation of pain, for example as a result of waiting to have a dressing changed (Soon and Acton 2006). Thus, pain, or anticipation of pain associated with treatment itself, may have detrimental effects on the process of chronic wound healing (see Fig. 3.1). In a series of studies Upton and colleagues suggested a link between pain, stress and healing in those with a chronic wound (e.g. Upton 2011a, b; Solowiej et al. 2009, 2010a, b). In particular, the evidence suggested that the stress of dressing change was a significant factor in those with a chronic wound.

This overview has indicated that stress may have an important part to play in both acute and chronic wound healing and hence it is important for the practitioner to be aware of stress, its definition and measurement and the potential impact it has on healing along with potential remediation strategies. Although there are many complex models of stress, there are two fundamental theories: The General Adaptation Syndrome (GAS) and the Interactional Model. These will be explored next since they underpin some of the subsequent observations and interventions in wound care.

General Adaption Syndrome (GAS) Model of Stress

The physiological model of stress- the General Adaption Syndrome (GAS) was proposed by Selye (1956). When a patient is experiencing stress there are usually a number of common bodily responses that can be identified, including; increased respiration, blood pressure or heart rate. These responses are all part of the 'fight or flight' syndrome that prepares the body and which are mediated through the nervous and endocrine system. The GAS describes three stages that are evident within the stress process, consisting of: (1) Alarm stage; (2) Resistance stage; (3) Exhaustion stage:

- **Alarm stage**: whereby the body prepares for the stressor by mobilising its available resources. This stage echo's that of the 'fight or flight' response in that the body's resources are mobilised for action. Nonetheless, if the stressor is persistent, resources become depleted leading to fatigue and subsequently triggers the resistance stage.
- **Resistance stage**: here the body adapts to the stressor, allowing physiological arousal to decline but still remaining higher than normal. It is here that the individual becomes at risk of health implications due to impaired immune functioning. Consequently, the exhaustion stage is triggered.

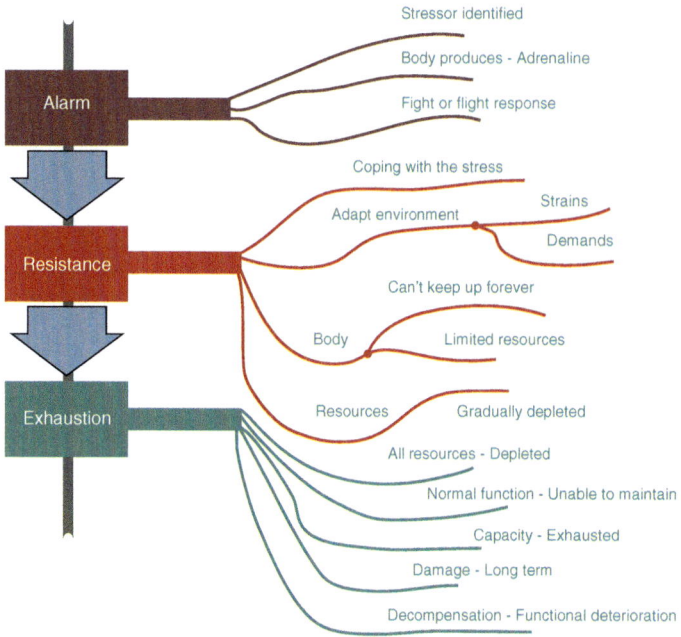

FIGURE 3.2 Model of the general adaption syndrome

- **Exhaustion stage**: When an individual's body is no longer able to respond and recover and resistance are no longer possible, a state of exhaustion will occur. This stage is highly detrimental and can lead to death.

The GAS was one of the first models of stress, being underpinned by the classic work of Cannon (1932): revealing that when an individual is stressed, physiological systems are activated in order to prepare for 'fight of flight' (Kemeny 2003). Although this process is beneficial to the individual in the short term, it can become highly maladaptive if the stressor becomes long term. Selye (1956), on the basis of the 'fight or flight' response, observed a number of animals and their reaction to stressful situations, discovering that this reaction was the beginning of a series of responses made by the body and ultimately physiological collapse, or exhaustion (see Fig. 3.2).

This prolonged experience of stress can significantly lower the immune functioning and the lower levels of various inflammatory cytokines and enzymes that are influential in tissue repair (Upton 2011a, b), and in the case of wound care, delayed wound healing. Such changes in cytokine and enzyme levels could explain the relationship between reduced wound healing and stress (Marucha et al. 1998). Physiologically, prolonged stress can lead to raised levels of the hormone cortisol. Although stress isn't the only reason that cortisol is secreted into the bloodstream, it has been termed "the stress hormone" because it is secreted in higher levels during the body's 'fight or flight' response to stress (Ebrecht et al. 2004). Higher and more prolonged levels of cortisol in the bloodstream have been shown to have negative effects on the body including, increased heart rate, higher blood pressure and lowered immunity and inflammatory responses in the body.

Psychologically, stress can increase the likelihood of patients making cognitive errors or negative appraisals, for example perceiving a dressing removal as an unpleasant experience, which can result in detrimental effects to the wound healing process and/or avoidance of treatment. Thus negative emotional responses affect biological and behavioural responses which feed back to further negatively affect the emotional response to pain, producing a continuous cycle (Adams et al. 2006) with delayed wound healing as a consequence. It is important for clinicians to recognise that pain and stress are both comprised of complex interactions between physiological, psychological and social factors (see Table 3.1).

Although the GAS model provided an insight into the physiological stress process, it regards the individual as responding to a stressor, with stress being a linear stimulus-response framework. In doing so it ignores the role of psychological factors and individual differences. Hence, Lazarus and Folkman (1984, 1987) developed an alternative model that integrated the potential for psychological variables: the interactional model of stress.

TABLE 3.1 Examples of psychological, biological and social factors contributing to both stress and pain

Psychological factors	Biological factors	Social factors
Negative emotional associations (e.g. anticipation of pain at dressing change)	Fight or flight response – sympathetic arousal	Availability and quality of social support
Previous experience of pain and stress	Cortisol released	Quality of personal relationships
Individual differences in perception/appraisal of a stressful event	Increase in heart rate, breathing rate, blood pressure	Social comparisons with other patients at different stages of recovery
Coping strategies	Lowered immune system functioning	Environmental factors (e.g. hospital/clinic attendance vs. home visits)

Interactional Model of Stress

Within the interactional model of stress, Lazarus and Folkman (1984, 1987) posited that stress and stress perception was based upon a transaction between an individual and their external world/environment. Hence, a stressful event would only elicit a stress response if the individual actually perceived the event to be stressful. In doing so, this model accounts for the individual differences that may be evident in perceiving an event stressful (E.g. while one patient may perceive a dressing change to be highly stressful, another may perceive it as a usual occurrence; see Fig. 3.3).

As can be seen in Fig. 3.3, this model proposes two types of appraisal; primary and secondary. The primary appraisal, whereby the event is appraised as to whether it is a threat or not (see Rovira et al. 2010a, b; Schlotz et al. 2011), is the initial

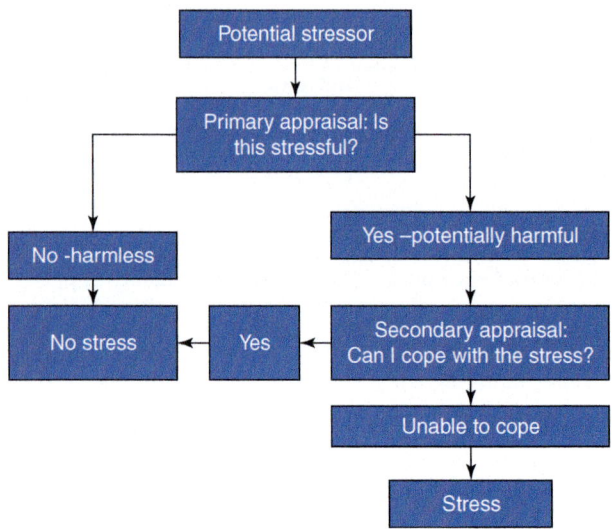

Figure 3.3 The interactional model of stress (Based on Lazarus and Folkman (1984, 1987))

response to a particular demand. From this, then two possible outcomes are available: either a threat or not (and the latter may either be positive, or neutral). If an individual perceives the situation to be threatening, secondary appraisal occurs; where the individual's ability to cope and the resources available are assessed (see Prati et al. 2010) and put into action. The available choices from this assessment reflects the control that the patient may have; taking control of the situation themself, gaining help from another, or avoiding the situation (this can be particularly influential when considering patient's treatment concordance, discussed later in this book). When an individual believes that, given their secondary appraisal, they have limited resources to cope with the situation, they will experience some form of stress and ultimately negative physiological consequences.

From this description of the model, a number of considerations for the wound care clinician can be noted. Firstly, clinicians cannot simply characterise a situation as stressful or not. Due to the differences in stress perception it may be that while one patient perceives a routine visit from the tissue viability nurse as stressful, another may perceive it as benign (or indeed, positive). Similarly, although the nurse may consider the dressing change as routine, normal and hence benign, the patient may not share this view. Furthermore, a patient whom may have experienced a previous painful experience during dressing removal may become highly stressed and anxious: their appraisal is based on learnt behaviour. Therefore, it is necessary for clinicians to be aware of such situations and consider patients on an individual basis.

Something which the clinician may view as routine clinical practice may be considered highly stressful by a patient (Upton 2011a, b). Secondly, the interactional model is based upon cognitive appraisal and is influenced by other psychological factors. Hence, it is possible for a patient to interpret the same situation in a number of differing ways depending on their mood- their cognitive appraisal is modified by their emotional state. Finally, it is important to remember that a patient can experience a stressful response irrespective of whether the event was experienced, anticipated or imagined. Within this model, the mere thought of having a dressing change itself can be stressful for the patient (Upton 2011a, b).

Lazarus and Folkman (1984) suggested two predominant functions of coping; the alteration of the situation (problem-focused coping), or regulation of emotional responses to the situation (emotional-focused coping). Briefly, problem-focused coping aims to reduce the stressful demands of expanding resources associated with dealing with that demand (e.g. this could include avoidance of dressing changes due to the stress perceived beforehand and during the procedure, or adopting a distraction strategy in order to help deal with the perceived stress). Alternatively, emotional-focused coping aims to regulate the emotional response through behavioural coping or cognitive coping strategies. For example, trying to stay calm throughout the treatment and reducing their own stress or worry.

Assessing Stress

It is well documented that psychological stress can result in delayed wound healing (Broadbent et al. 2003; Ebrecht et al. 2004; Francis and Pennebaker 1992; Gouin et al. 2008; Jones et al. 2006; Marucha et al. 1998; Weinman et al. 2008). Also, as highlighted previously in this chapter, stress can result in distorted cognition and subsequent increased pain. Hence, it is essential for wound care professionals to assess patient's psychological stress throughout the treatment regime. Self-report or physiological measures should be used to assess patient's stress in addition to an awareness of patient's behavioural (see Table 3.2) indicators of stress.

In order for clinicians to assess levels of stress and pain in patients with chronic wounds, it is important to recognise that both stress and pain are biopsychosocial concepts (i.e. both stress and pain are comprised of complex interactions between biological, psychological and social components) and hence both physiological and psychological measures are required.

Effective psychological measures of stress focus upon the emotional responses obtained through self-report methods (see Table 3.3 for brief overview). Self-report methods of measuring stress are common in investigating patients' response to illness/injury (e.g. chronic wounds) and can range from a simple "stress-thermometer" (for example, see Fig. 3.4) to more formal psychometric measures. For example, the PSS

Table 3.2 Behavioural signs of stress
Rapid breathing rate.
Faster eye-blink rate.
Increased heart rate.
Muscle tension.
Squirming, sweating palms.
Dry mouth, tense voice.
Pale skin, cold sweat.
Avoidance behaviour.

TABLE 3.3 An evaluation of a selection of psychological measures of stress

Measure	Purpose	Strengths	Weaknesses
The Hospital Anxiety and Depression Scale (HADS), (Zigmond and Snaith 1983)	Designed for use in medical out-patient clinics to detect clinical cases of anxiety and depression and to assess the severity of anxiety and depression.	Measures state anxiety and depression in a specific clinical setting. Short scale (14-items), that takes approx 10 min for the patient to complete.	Items are designed to measure state anxiety rather than stress. However, anxiety is an outcome of stress.
The State Trait Anxiety Inventory (STAI), (Spielberger 1977)	Designed to measure state and trait anxiety in adults. Clearly differentiates the temporary condition of "state anxiety" and the more general long-term "trait anxiety".	The state aspect of the questionnaire can determine anxiety in a specific situation (i.e. at dressing change) rather than in a more general sense. It can be used with clinical patients. Includes a 40-item scale which takes approx 10 min to complete.	

(continued)

TABLE 3.3 (continued)

Measure	Purpose	Strengths	Weaknesses
The Perceived Stress Scale (PSS), (Cohen and Hoberman 1983)	Designed to measure the degree to which situations in a person's life are perceived as stressful. Higher scores indicate more perceived stress.	The PSS is more successful in predicting a variety of health and health care outcomes than measures of life events which focus on the number rather than the appraisal of the events.	This questionnaire includes items that refer to "the last month". In terms of assessing stress levels specific to chronic wounds at dressing changes, this measure is more general.
The General Health Questionnaire (GHQ), (Goldberg et al. 1978)	Designed to detect non-psychotic psychiatric disorder in people in community and medical settings. Higher scores indicate greater emotional distress.	The GHQ-28 version assesses anxiety, insomnia and severe depression. Identifies individuals' health behaviours.	This questionnaire is not a measure of psychological stress; however it can be used to accompany other measures of stress to provide information on health behaviours.

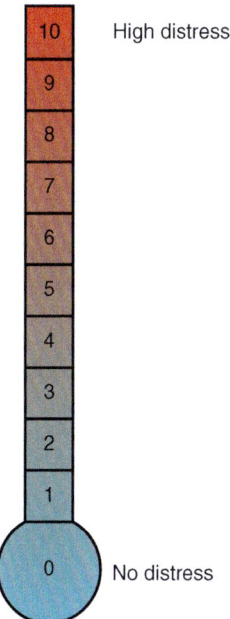

FIGURE 3.4 Stress thermometer

allows clinicians to assess a patient's psychological appraisal of stress, whereas a measurement of increased heart rate or blood pressure would show a physiological outcome of stress. Accurate assessments of this nature allow us to determine the impact of interventions on psychological stress and anxiety in such situations. An overview of some of the more popular psychological measures of stress is presented here.

The Perceived Stress Scale (PSS; Cohen 1983)

The PSS was developed to measure patients perceptions of how stressful particular situations in their left were, with high scores indicating higher perceived stress. Rather than being focused on the number of stressful events patient's experience, the PSS placed emphasis on the patient's appraisal of the stressful events. Despite this, the PSS is a more general measure of stress in that it refers to occurrences of stress related thoughts and feelings which have been experienced over the previous month. Thus, this measure may render inapplicable when considering stress induced in specific clinical situations (i.e. during dressing changes).

The State Trait Anxiety Inventory (STAI; Speilberger 1977)

This particular measure differs to that discussed above in that it can measure stress in relation to a specific clinical situation (i.e. during dressing changes). It is designed in order to differentiate between a temporary condition of state of anxiety and long term experience of train anxiety. Due to this, the STAI can be advantageous to the clinician in terms of wound assessments.

The General Health Questionnaire (GHQ; Goldberg et al. 1978)

This particular method was developed in order to measure emotional distress presented in patients within both community and clinical settings, with higher scores indicating higher emotional distress. The GHQ items are also designed to identify patient's health behaviours. One particular advantage of this measure is its emphasis on measuring anxiety, insomnia and depression but without placing a focus on physical symptoms of illness. Although the GHQ can be used in conjunction with other measures of stress, its items are not specifically designed to measure patient stress. Thus, it may not be applicable when implemented within a wound-care regime alone.

The Hospital Anxiety and Depression Scale (HADS; Zigmond and Snaith 1983)

Finally, the HADS, a 14-item scale, was developed to assess clinical cases of anxiety and depression in medical out-patient settings. As with the other measures, higher score indicated greater anxiety or depression. This measure can be particularly advantageous to the wound health professional in that it can be implemented at intervals in order to assess any differences which may be apparent over time (i.e. such as before, during and after dressing changes).

The assessment and re-assessment of patient's experiences of pain and stress, using these tools or similar, should be an essential aspect of wound care and management (Freedman et al. 2003). Failure to assess pain and stress can lead to considerable distress for the patient, not only during treatment but also the period before treatment, due to the emotive responses associated with anticipation of the painful experience (Soon and Acton 2006). Hence, appropriate and consistent assessment of such pain can equip clinicians with the understanding necessary in administering suitable methods of pain relief (Upton and Solowiej 2010). Additionally, accurate assessment and management of pain can lead to significant reductions in patient's psychological stress. Hence, in order to fully facilitate wound healing, it is important for health professionals to assess both pain and stress (Tables 3.3 and 3.4).

However, using individual measures of psychological stress alone can be problematic. The use of a single self-report method to assess a patient's level of psychological stress could be subject to biases such as social desirability and/or demand characteristics (for example, patients might believe they should report higher levels of psychological stress in order to meet the expectations of the clinician).

There are also a number of physiological measures of stress that are commonly used when assessing patients' stress levels, which can be beneficial as physiological responses are innate and are shielded from biases that self-report measures are subjected to, such as demand characteristics. However, physiological measures alone do not necessarily confirm the presence of psychological stress, for example, an increase in heart rate or blood pressure could be due to any number of factors, and not just psychological stress. Table 3.4 shows a number of methods that can be used to measure patients' physiological responses to stress.

TABLE 3.4 An evaluation of a selection of physiological measures of stress

Measure	Purpose	Strengths	Weaknesses
Saliva sampling to assess levels of cortisol	To measure the levels of cortisol present in saliva. Higher levels of cortisol indicate greater reported psychological stress.	Self-collection pack can be provided to patients to take their own swabs at specific times during the day. Cortisol levels can be correlated with the speed of wound healing.	This method should accompany other measures of stress to eliminate other possible causes of elevated cortisol levels.
Actigraphy: Actiwatch monitoring system	A wrist-worn motor activity monitor which measures human rest/activity cycles.	Useful for determining sleep cycles/sleep disruption.	Not a measure of psychological stress. Problematic to determine a clear link between sleep disruption and psychological stress as a result of chronic wounds.
Blood Pressure	Elevated blood pressure is a physiological symptom associated with the body's stress response.	Blood pressure measurements can be taken at intervals before, during and after activity, such as dressing change.	Measures of elevated blood pressure alone do not solely determine levels of psychological stress as this may be due to other factors.

TABLE 3.4 (continued)

Measure	Purpose	Strengths	Weaknesses
Heart Rate	Elevated heart rate is a physiological symptom associated with the body's stress response.	Heart rate can be monitored at intervals before, during and after activity, such as dressing change.	Measures of increased heart rate alone do not solely determine levels of psychological stress as this may be due to other factors.
GSR (Galvanic Skin Response)	A method of measuring the electrical resistance of the skin. Increased GSR is a physiological symptom associated with the body's stress response.	GSR can be measured at intervals before, during and after activity, such as dressing change.	Measures of increased GSR alone do not solely determine levels of psychological stress as this may be due to other factors.

Relationship Between Stress, Pain and Wound Healing

A number of studies have reported on the link between stress and wound healing in both clinical and non-clinical populations and in both acute and chronic wounds. For example, when 11 dental students received biopsy wounds on the palate of their mouth (the first being administered during their summer vacation and the second, before term examinations), photographs and foaming response to hydrogen peroxide were used to examine wound healing (Marucha et al. 1998). It was discovered that wounds administered during the stressful period (i.e. the students' examinations) took approximately 40 % longer (an average of 3 days) to heal. Additionally, indicating the possibility of one immunological mechanism, during the stress period, production of interleukin-1 beta declined significantly (68 %). Moreover, Ebrecht et al. (2004) examined the relationship between perceived stress and wound healing. After receiving a 4 mm biopsy wound, participants were monitored using ultrasound scanning. The Perceived Stress Scale (PSS; Cohen et al. 1983) and the General Health Questionnaire (GHQ-12; Goldberg 1992) were also administered to participants in order to account for stress and health behaviours. Finally, cortisol assessments were conducted on participant's saliva samples. It was discovered that as PSS and GHQ-12 scores increased, speed of wound healing decreased. Additionally, cortisol assessments from the morning following the biopsy negatively correlated with speed of wound healing. It was concluded that the implications of perceived stress are quite substantial in wound healing.

Other research has explored psychological stress in more ecologically valid studies. For example, biopsy wounds have been administered to 13 women caring for relatives with Alzheimer's disease and a control group in order to assess wound healing (Kiecolt-Glaser et al. 1995). In addition to the completion of the PSS at the time of biopsy and 1 week later, wounds were photographed and assessed using hydrogen peroxide. Findings highlighted the negative associated between stress and wound healing with caregivers reporting more stress and their wounds taking approximated 9 days longer to heal. Hence, it is apparent from the above study that in addition to stressful experiences, chronic stress can significantly impact upon a patient's wound healing. This, and the previous studies, are influential in providing clinicians with a foundation to the importance of the relationship between stress and wound healing. However, in order to apply such understanding to the complex nature of wound care, it is also essential to explore this stress-wound relationship in relation to patients with naturally occurring chronic wounds.

Much research has indicated a link between stress and delayed wound healing in chronic wounds (Cole-King and Harding 2001; Soon and Acton 2006; Walburn et al. 2009; Solowiej et al. 2009, 2010a, b). Walburn et al. (2009) and Solowiej et al. (2009), in their respective reviews of the scientific literature reported that stress was associated with delayed wound healing in older adults, particularly those suffering with leg wounds and surgical patients. There is consequently evidence from both lab studies and in the clinical setting that stress delays healing. However, just as importantly- can reducing stress improve healing? One such study has explored whether a traditional stress-reducing intervention can improve healing. A study considering the effect of an emotional disclosure intervention on biopsy wound patients emphasised the positive impact of minimising stress on wound healing (Weinman et al. 2008).

Although the above findings illustrate the importance of reducing stress in relation to biopsy and surgical wounds, they cannot be applied to that of chronic wounds. It would be presumptuous, particularly given the lack of exploratory research, to assume that such findings would be illustrative of the stress-chronic wound relationship, particularly as chronic wound may not necessarily follow the same healing process (Solowiej et al. 2009). Thus, wound–care professionals also need to consider the studies that provide support for the negative consequences of stress upon wound healing. For example, the relationship between anxiety, depression and chronic wound healing has been investigated by Cole-King and Harding (2001). Patient's depression and anxiety were measured using the Hospital Anxiety and Depression Scale (HADS; Zigmond and Snaith 1983) while also rating their healing via a 5-point Likert scale. A statistically significant relationship was discovered with higher HADS scores being associated with delayed wound healing. Similar findings were reported by Jones et al. (2006) who suggest that pain and odour were the two most influential symptoms. Hence, such stress management interventions are essential within clinical wound-care practice. Not only could stress increase incidence, but also reoccurrence of chronic wounds (Norman 2003). The implementation of interventions can benefit the healing process, while, in some instances, also reduce distress and improve quality of life (Upton 2011a, b).

As discussed earlier, research has highlighted the significant impact of psychological stress on wound healing, with further research suggesting a link between stress and increased pain sensitivity (Leistad et al. 2006). However, there is limited research available elucidating the link between pain and stress in chronic wound patients (Upton 2011a, b). Research conducted by Upton and colleagues (2011a, b) has explored the link between pain and stress at dressing change. Pain and stress were recorded (using psychological and physiological measures) from 39 patients at baseline and during dressing change. Significant differences were discovered between baseline and dressing change responses for heart rate, pain rating, stress rating and anxiety. Furthermore, all measurements indicated higher scores during dressing chance, highlighting increased pain and stress. Additionally, it was discovered that chronic stress correlated with stress at dressing change and pain at dressing change. Based upon these results, it could be concluded that chronic stress levels impact upon pain and stress intensity during dressing change (Leistad et al. 2006), or that continual, regular experiences of pain and stress caused by the wound and dressing chance contributes to chronic stress (see Fig. 3.5).

In a similar study to those conducted by Upton's team (e.g. Upton et al. 2013a, b; Upton and Solowiej 2010, 2012; Upton and South 2012; Upton et al. 2012a, b, c; Solowiej and Upton 2010a, b), Parvaneh et al. (2014) reported that patients visiting a DFU clinic experienced stress when attending the clinic. Using a novel and innovative recording technique, the use of wearable stress-monitors allowed for the physiological consequences of stress to be recorded on a real-time basis. The study reported that the highest stressful condition was during wound dressing change, which was related to either the pain or painful dressing. Again, confirming other studies (Upton and Solowiej 2012) that suggests minimising pain and stress

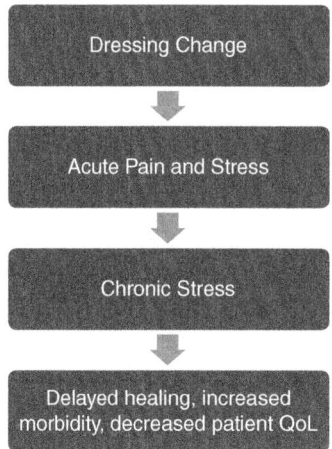

FIGURE 3.5 A potential relationship between pain and stress at dressing change and delayed wound healing (Upton 2011a, b)

at wound dressing change may prove beneficial to the patient and their wound healing.

Ebrecht et al. (2004) highlight the negative consequences of patients living with chronic stress, including that of increased cortisol. Not only does this hormone negatively impact immunity but, can lead to delayed wound healing, subsequent reduction in quality of life and increased chronic stress. Clinicians need to acknowledge the cumulative impact of the stress frequently perceived at dressing change. In doing so, professionals need to consider the selection of appropriate dressing as this may decrease the pain and stress at dressings. In addition, the clinician should also consider the range of stress management techniques that may be available.

Stress Management

When an individual experiences stress, fear or anxiety, the pain pathways become more sensitised than when a patient is calm and fear-free. Hence, a patient's psychological state can influence their experience of pain. Stress can have a significant impact on the way in which a patient perceives pain, with research highlighting high stress and pain anticipation as resulting in the experience of increased pain intensity (Solowiej et al. 2009; Upton et al. 2012a,). Therefore, it is reasonable to conclude that heightened stress and anxiety can, as previously noted, result in a lowered pain threshold and reduced pain tolerance (Woo et al. 2009).

Due to the detrimental impact of stress upon pain and wound healing, it is essential for health professionals to adopt some form of 'stress management techniques' in order to minimise or manage its occurrence (Upton 2011a, b). A number of such methods have been developed in order to try and reduce or teach patient's to cope with their stress some of which will be outlined below.

Managing Stressors

Firstly, in order to reduce stress it is necessary to remove, if at all possible, the stressor or modify the exposure to stressful situations. However, achieving this with stressors related to patients with chronic wounds can prove difficult. For instance, wound related stressors such as dressing changes cannot be 'removed' due to its essential element in the treatment of wounds. If patients were to avoid such essential elements of wound care, negative physical consequences may arise (this will be discussed later in the book). Alternatively, rather than remove the stressor (i.e. the dressing change), it may be more appropriate for the clinician to modify the technique used.

Research has highlighted a number of wound dressings that can cause pain and tissue trauma during the dressing change procedure. These include alginate, foam, film, hydrogel, and hydrocolloid (Hollinworth and Collier 2000). The pain experienced during the use of one of these dressings can result in the patient experiencing heightened stress and subsequent pain. Thus, a more appropriate dressing which facilitates reduction in pain and trauma should be considered as an alternative technique, thereby modifying the stressful situation. These may involve the use of soft silicone which adheres without damaging the fragile tissue of the wound. Hence, clinicians substituting one of the dressings noted above with ones utilising newer technologies can significantly reduce and sometimes prevent the occurrence of pain and wound trauma of their patients (Dykes et al. 2001; Dykes 2007; White 2008; WUWHS 2007). Subsequently, the patient's perceived anxiety and stress would reduce resulting in the disruption of the pain-stress-pain cycle.

Sometimes it is possible to get the patient to reappraise the situation. When a stressor cannot avoid a particular stressor it may be beneficial to get the patient to focus more on the positive aspects of their wound management, such as improved health and removed pain. This approach is often adopted in cognitive behavioural interventions and has been discovered to be useful to the wound-healing process. Similarly, it may be beneficial to teach patients coping techniques such as relaxation, active wound management and reappraisal. This could also include the promotion of social support (see Chap. 7), through sharing and discussing emotions and experiences with other patients.

A number of techniques have been adopted in promoting relaxation including Progressive Muscle Relaxation (PMR). This relaxation technique was developed by Jacobson (1938) and proposed that the determining mechanism for relaxation was the patient's ability to understand the difference between tension and relaxation. This ability to differentiate between the two is taught through the successive tensing and relaxing of a number of muscle groups.

Health care professionals can also influence a patient's perceived pain and stress through effective communicating with their patients (Chap. 8). Furthermore, clinicians can ensure that the environment in which the wound treatment is conducted is calm throughout the procedure. Visual imagery can also assist the alleviation of pain with clinicians guiding the imagery (i.e. asking patients to imagine they are on a beach, listening to the breeze, or even imagining they are at a football game). Distraction can also assist in reducing pain by asking the patient to do something that will require concentration (such as doing multiplications). As their concentration is directed towards the multiplication the pain they perceive during treatment will be lessened (Upton 2011a, b).

Conclusion

The studies above add to an expanding evidence base supporting the link between stress, pain and delayed wound healing. The discovery that stress and pain experienced during wound healing can negatively impact upon the total healing period has significant implications for clinical practice. It is essential that clinicians assess such stress and pain in order to manage it appropriately, subsequently, resulting in improved wound repair. Additionally, such assessments need to be based upon the needs of individual patients in order to offer the more effective treatment and mode of care. Measurements need to include both psychological and physiological measures; with clinicians monitoring physiological processes whilst also communicating with patients, acknowledging their feedback on perceived stress. In this way, treatments can be modified and appropriate stress-management processes put in place.

References

Adams N, Poole H, Richardson C. Psychological approaches to chronic pain management. J Clin Nurs. 2006;15:290–300.

Broadbent E, Petrie KJ, Alley PG, et al. Psychological stress impairs early wound repair following surgery. Psychosom Med. 2003;65: 865–9.

Cannon WB. The wisdom of the body. New York: Norton; 1932.

Cohen S, Hoberman H. Positive events and social supports as buffers of life change stress. J Appl Soc Psychol. 1983;13:99–125.

Cohen S, Karmarck T, Mermelstein R. A global measure of perceived stress. J Health Soc Behav. 1983;24:385–96.

Cole-King A, Harding KG. Psychological factors and delayed healing in chronic wounds. Psychosom Med. 2001;63:216–20.

Dykes PJ. The effect of adhesive dressing edges on cutaneous irritancy and skin barrier function. J Wound Care. 2007;16(3):97–100.

Dykes PJ, Heggie R, Hill SA. Effects of adhesive dressings on the stratum corneum of the skin. J Wound Care. 2001;10(2):7–10.

Ebrecht M, Hextall J, Kirtley LG, Taylor A, Dyson M, Weinman J. Perceived stress and cortisol levels predict speed of wound healing in healthy male adults. Psychoneuroendocrinology. 2004; 29(6):798–809.

Francis ME, Pennebaker JW. Putting stress into words: writing about personal upheavals and health. Am J Health Promot. 1992;6:280–7.

Freedman G, Cean C, Duron V, et al. Pathogenesis and treatment of pain in patients with chronic wounds. Surg Technol Int. 2003;11: 168–79.

Glaser R, Kiecolt-Glaser JK, Marucha PT, et al. Stress-related changes in pro-inflammatory cytokine production in wounds. Arch Gen Psychiatry. 1999;56:450–6.

Goldberg LR. The development of markers for the Big-Five factor structure. Psychol Assess. 1992;4:26–42.

Goldberg DP, et al. Manual of the general health questionnaire. England: Windsor; 1978.

Gouin JP, Kiecolt-Glaser JK, Malarkey WB, Glaser R. The influence of anger expression on wound healing. Brain Behav Immun. 2008; 22:699–708.

Hollinworth H, Collier M. Nurses' views about pain and trauma at dressing changes: results of a national survey. J Wound Care. 2000; 9(8):369–73.

Jacobson E. Progressive muscle relaxation. Chicago: University of Chicago Press; 1938.

Jones J, Barr W, Robinson J, Carlisle C. Depression in patients with chronic venous ulceration. Br J Nurs. 2006;15(11):17–23.

Kemeny ME. The psychology of stress. Curr Dir Psychol Sci. 2003;12(4):124–9.

Kiecolt-Glaser JK, Marucha PT, Malarkey WB, Mercado AM, Glaser R. Slowing of wound healing by psychological stress. Lancet. 1995;346:1194–6.

Lazarus RS, Folkman S. Stress, appraisal, and coping. New York: Springer; 1984.

Lazarus RS, Folkman S. Transactional theory and research on emotions and coping. Eur J Pers. 1987;1(3):141–69.

Leistad RB, Sand T, Westgaard RH, Nilsen KB, Stovner LJ. Stress-induced pain and muscle activity in patients with migraine and tension-type headache. Cephalalgia. 2006;26(1):64–73.

Marucha PT, Kiecolt-Glaser JK, Favagehis M. Muscol wound healing is impaired by examination stress. Psychosom Med. 1998;60(3): 362–5.

Norman D. The effects of stress on wound healing and leg ulceration. Br J Nurs. 2003;12:1256–63.

Parvaneh S, Grewal GS, Grewal E, Menzies RA, Talal TK, Armstrong DG, Sternberg E, Najafi B. Stressing the dressing: assessing stress during wound care in real-time using wearable sensors. Wound Med. 2014;4:21–6.

Prati G, Pietrontoni L, Cicognani E. Self-efficacy moderates the relationship between stress appraisal and quality of life among rescue workers. Anxiety Stress Coping. 2010;23(4):463–70.

Rovira M, Scott SG, Liss AS, Jensen J, Thayer SP, Leach SD. Isolation and characterization of centroacinar/terminal ductal progenitor cells in adult mouse pancreas. Natl Acad Sci. 2010a;107:75–80.

Rovira T, Edo S, Fernandez-Castro J. How does cognitive appraisal lead to perceived stress in academic examinations. Stud Psychol. 2010b;52(3):179–92.

Schlotz W, Hammefald K, Ehlert U, Gaab J. Individual differences in the cortisol response to stress in young healthy men: testing the roles of perceived stress reactivity and threat appraisal using multiphase latent growth curve modelling. Biol Psychol. 2011;87(2): 257–64.

Selye H. What is stress? Metabolism. 1956;5(5):525–30.

Solowiej K, Upton D. Take it easy: how the cycle of stress and pain associated with wound care affects recovery. Nurs Residential Care. 2010a;12(9):443–6.

Solowiej K, Upton D. The assessment and management of pain and stress in wound care. Br J Community Nurs. 2010b;15(6):S26–33.

Solowiej K, Mason V, Upton D. Review of the relationship between stress and wound healing: part 1. J Wound Care. 2009;18(9):357–66.

Solowiej K, Mason V, Upton D. Psychological stress and pain in wound care, part 3: management. J Wound Care. 2010a;19(4):153–5.

Solowiej K, Mason V, Upton D. Psychological stress and pain in wound care, part 2: a review of pain and stress assessment tools. J Wound Care. 2010b;19(3):110–5.

Soon K, Acton C. Pain-induced stress: a barrier to wound healing. Wounds UK. 2006;2(4):92–101.

Spielberger CD. Anxiety: theory and research. In: Wolman BB, editor. International encyclopedia of neurology, psychiatry, psychoanalysis and psychology. New York: Human Sciences Press; 1977. p. 81–4.

Upton D. Psychological impact of pain in patients with wounds. London: Wounds UK; 2011a.

Upton D. Psychology of stress. In: Upton D, editor. Psychological impact of pain in patients with wounds. London: Wounds UK; 2011b.

Upton D, Solowiej K. Pain and stress as contributors to delayed wound healing. Wound Pract Res. 2010;18(3):114–22.

Upton D, Solowiej K. The impact of a traumatic vs conventional dressings on pain and stress. J Wound Care. 2012;21(5):209–15.

Upton D, South F. The Psychological consequences of wounds- a vicious circle that should not be overlooked. Wounds UK. 2012;7(4):116–8.

Upton D, Solowiej K. Using electronic voting systems in wound care conferences. Wounds UK. 2011;7(1):58–61.

Upton D, Hender C, Solowiej K. Mood disorders in patients with acute and chronic wounds: a health professional perspective. J Wound Care. 2012a;21(1):42–8.

Upton D, Hender C, Solowiej K, Woo K. Stress and pain associated with dressing change in chronic wound patients. J Wound Care. 2012b;22(2):53–61.

Upton D, Solowiej K, Hender C, Woodyat KY. Stress and pain associated with dressing change in patients with chronic wounds. J Wound Care. 2012c;21(2):53–61.

Upton D, Morgan J, Andrews A, et al. The pain and stress of wound treatment in patients with burns. An international burn specialist perspective. Wounds. 2013a;25(8):199–204.

Upton D, Stephens D, Andrews A. Patients' experience of negative pressure wound therapy. J Wound Care. 2013b;22(1):34–9.

Walburn J, Vedhara K, Hankins M, Rixon L, Weinman J. Psychological stress and wound healing in humans: a systematic review and meta-analysis. J Psychosom Res. 2009;67:253–71.

Weinman J, Ebrecht M, Scott S, Walburn J, Dyson M. Enhanced wound healing after emotional disclosure intervention. Br J Health Psychol. 2008;13:95–102.

White R. A multinational survey of the assessment of pain when removing dressings. Wounds UK. 2008;4(1):1–6.

Woo KY, Coutts PM, Price P, Harding K, Sibbald RG. A randomized crossover investigation of pain at dressing change comparing 2 foam dressings. Adv Skin Wound Care. 2009;22(7):304–10.

World Union of Wound Healing Societies. Principles of best practice: wound exudate and the role of dressings. A consensus document. London: MEP; 2007.

Zigmond AS, Snaith RP. The hospital anxiety & depression scale. Acta Psychiatr Scand. 1983;67:361–70.

Chapter 4
Quality of Life and Well-Being

> Box 4.1: Key Points
> - Quality of life and well-being are umbrella terms that refer to an individual's subjective ratings of their satisfaction with life, and affective state respectively;
> - Despite being widely used, these terms are poorly defined and often misused; for example, although often used interchangeably, quality of life and well-being are not synonyms, nor are they on the same continuum;
> - Health related quality of life is an important patient reported outcome that measures the (negative) impact of the wound and treatment strategies on daily functioning and mental health (deficit model);
> - In contrast well-being assesses the presence of positive psychological variables that may protect the patient's mental health (resource model);
> - Assessment currently focuses on the deficit model, however this is limited, as the absence of mental health problems should not be taken to indicate good well-being;

> - Given what we already know about psychological health, increasing the focus on well-being may provide a mechanism through which to boost a patient's psychological resources thereby reducing anxiety, stress and pain, and accelerate the healing process.

Summary

The assessment of quality of life (QoL) has become progressively important over the past 25 years. In clinical settings this is usually called health related quality of life (HRQoL), which has become well-established as an essential patient reported outcome measure (PROM). A related concept, which is garnering increasing interest, is subjective well-being. Despite some commonalities, HRQoL and well-being should be treated as separate concepts; they should not be used as synonyms. In short, HRQoL refers to the cognitive appraisal which a patient makes about the impact their health has on their daily life, whilst well-being concerns a patient's emotional response to their wound, its treatment and their future. This chapter explores these concepts in more detail, beginning by explaining the theoretical foundations of QoL and wellbeing, and describing the conceptual models that can be applied to wound care. Ways of measuring QoL and well-being are also discussed, before finally the implications for practice, and the benefits for patient care are determined.

Introduction

Researchers and health care professionals place great importance on the improvement and maintenance of the QoL and well-being of chronically ill patients (Herber et al. 2007). Today QoL measures are routinely used to evaluate psychosocial and economic costs and benefits of various health

Introduction

interventions; indeed their inclusion as an outcome measure in randomised control trials (RCT) has become standard practice (Fayers and Machin 2007). This is in part a response to the recognition that whilst advances in medical science have enabled us to increase longevity, this is often at a cost. For example, many chronic wounds result from other long term conditions such as diabetes, vascular disease, obesity or spinal cord injury, as well as being a corollary of an aging population (Sen et al. 2009). Treatments may be aggressive, causing as much pain and distress as the illness itself. Furthermore, despite medical advancement it is not always possible to cure. Thus in palliative care, QoL is not just an outcome, but also an endpoint measure. In both cases, patient choice becomes a vital part of the clinical decision making process (Shukla et al. 2008). Wounds have variable, and often protracted healing rates, which can lead to a wound becoming chronic even when optimum care is being provided. Clinicians may therefore need to acknowledge early on in the care process that for some patients, whilst healing may be the main intended outcome in the longer term, it may not be the priority of care. Incorporating a measure of QoL and well-being within a care pathway, shifts the focus from the wound and physical outcomes such as healing, to the whole person, with the aim of making living with a wound the best it can be.

Despite the ubiquitous nature of QoL assessment in recent years, and the assimilation of terms such as well-being into common parlance, a lack of consensus remains in both academic and clinical settings, regarding the definitions of QoL and well-being. This has led in turn to the development of a range of models and approaches to assessing QoL and well-being. Consequently, negotiating this field can be bewildering to the uninitiated. The aim of this chapter is therefore to provide a clear summary of the dominant theories and measurement approaches in the field, before providing guidance to the application of this theory and measurement in practice, and the possible value for both clinicians and patients with wounds (See Box 4.1).

Theories of QoL and Wellbeing

QoL is a hypothetical construct that acts as 'an organising concept that exists to guide its users' (Wallander 2001). In other words it has no physical foundation, but is rather inferred from first-hand experience and theoretical knowledge. Given this definition, it is not surprising that it has been referred to as a 'vague, ethereal construct' (Shukla et al. 2008). It is also a concept that is applied widely from economics, through social policy to health. This wide application, coupled with its hypothetical foundations, also explains why there is such difficulty in agreeing a definition; definitions vary in part depending on the aspect of our daily lives to which QoL is being applied, and the perspective of the user. In fact it has been suggested that having multiple definitions is helpful from a theoretical perspective (Wallander 2001), as it allows users to actualise the definition which best suits their needs. Thus an economist, social policy maker and a clinician can work with the definitions that is most apt for their purposes. Well-being is also a very abstract concept, and like quality of life definitions are known to be both 'ambiguous' and nebulous' (Galloway et al. 2006). However, this is not helpful from an applied perspective, and so the aim of this section is to provide a useful working definition that can be employed in clinical practice.

QoL is a complex phenomenon that concerns an individual's satisfaction with all aspects of life from the physical to the social and psychological. It is affected by many factors including income, social and physical environment, interpersonal relationships and health. The World Health Organisation (WHO) defined QoL as:

> 'an individual's perception of their position in life in the context of the culture and value systems in which they live, and in relation to their goals, expectations, standards and concerns'(p1, WHO 1997)

Usually in health care settings the focus is on assessing the impact of changes in health status on a patient's QoL; this type of assessment is very specific and should be referred to

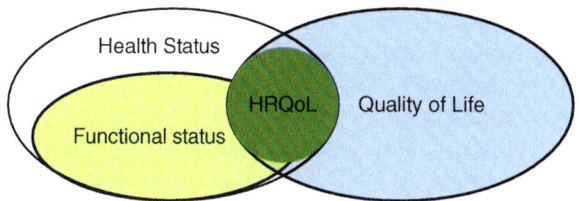

FIGURE 4.1 The relationship between QoL, HRQoL, functional status and health status (Based on Morrison et al. (2003))

as health related QoL or HRQoL. In practice however the terms QoL and HRQoL are often used interchangeably, although it can sometimes be useful to make the distinction between HRQoL and QoL.

HRQoL is itself a complex, multidimensional construct, which focuses on an individual's experience of the impact that their health status has on their QoL. HRQoL should not therefore be confused with either health status or functional status. Although these terms are also sometimes used interchangeably, this is conceptually inaccurate. Whilst it can be difficult to distinguishing these three concepts, it is not impossible. The difficulty lies in their shared characteristics. Health status refers to the evaluation (either objective or subjective) of a person's state of health including any illness, treatment and level of functioning; functional status is therefore a part of health status and indicates an individual's capacity to carry out everyday tasks (Morrison et al. 2003). This relationship is shown diagrammatically in Fig. 4.1.

Figure 4.1 also demonstrates, health status and functioning will impact to some extent on an individual's QoL. HRQoL therefore concerns the interface between an individual's health status, functioning and QoL and is therefore a distinct and specific component of QoL. Of course, since HRQoL is one aspect of our overall QoL, it is inevitable that changes in HRQoL will influence overall QoL. Thus whilst in a clinical setting the *measurement* may focus specifically on HRQoL, when considering the *impact* of having a chronic wound on the individual the distinction between HRQoL and QoL is less clear.

According to Draper and Thompson (2001), HRQoL is one of the most widely used terms in the health care profession, being applied across professions (nursing, allied health, health economists, public health) and activities (e.g. research, medical ethics, health services management). Despite this, there is no consensus on definition, even at this level of specificity. Different ways of conceptualizing HRQoL can therefore be found throughout the literature (Rapley 2003; Lach et al. 2006). As with QoL, definitions appear to depend upon the perspective and purpose of the clinician or researcher; for example, a surgeon is most likely to focus on HRQoL as a tool to assess health *outcomes* following life saving treatment, whereas an epidemiologist will want to assess the *determinants* of HRQoL.

Wellbeing is also sometimes used as a synonym for QoL, and again this is neither correct nor desirable. Well-being has been defined as:

> 'a holistic, subjective state which is present when a range of feelings, among them energy, confidence, openness, enjoyment, happiness, calm and caring are combined and balanced' (Pawlyn and Carnaby 2009)

Although QoL and well-being inevitably overlap – both are subjective assessments and both refer to psychological states – and the terms are often used interchangeably, it is important to distinguish between the two. In essence, QoL refers to a person's cognitive assessment of their overall standard of living, or their 'personal assessment of life satisfaction' (Price and Harding 2004). As can be seen from the WHO definition, QoL asks about an individual's perception of what their life is like. In contrast, the term 'well-being' refers to the presence of positive emotions and contentment, with the absence of long-lasting and persistent negative emotions (e.g. Zikmund 2003; CDC 2011). Well-being therefore refers to an individual's emotional response to what their life is like. In essence, QoL (and therefore HRQoL) concerns the cognitive appraisal of an individual's situation, whereas well-being refers to their emotional appraisal. This is a very clear

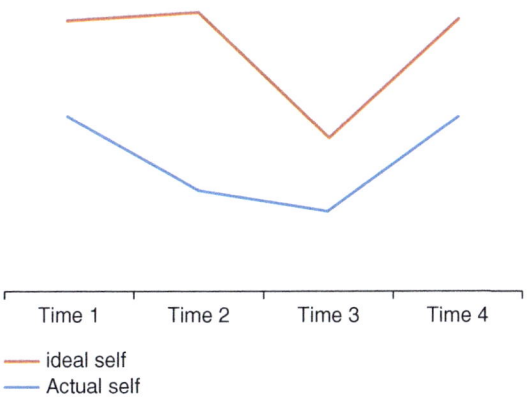

Figure 4.2 An illustration of gap theory

distinction, one that can help provide a useful working definition which can be applied in practice.

In summary, QoL is a broad concept, an umbrella term which encompasses HRQoL, and is related to well-being. As noted earlier, a number of factors impact upon our QoL including health, income, social status and of course our well-being. It is of course just as likely that our well-being is in turn influenced by these same factors – health, income, social status and QoL. It is therefore probably more accurate to view QoL and well-being as interdependent factors that work together in a dynamic relationship.

The relationship between well-being and QoL is undoubtedly a complex one. To begin to work this out, we first need to understand how individuals reach an assessment of their QoL. It is usually suggested that QoL is the gap between a person's expectations and their fulfilment. This is commonly known as 'gap theory' and is illustrated in Fig. 4.2. Thus it is assumed that poorer QoL is the result of discrepancies between an individual's actual ('like me') and ideal self ('how I would like to be') (Eiser and Eiser 2000). As Fig. 4.2 demonstrates this can fluctuate over time as functioning and expectations change. Figure 4.2 illustrates how a person's

QoL might fluctuate over time. Thus at Time 2 an event, such as diagnosis of a venous ulcer provokes a change in a person's perception of themselves, thus widening the gap between actual and ideal self and lowering QoL. At Time 3 the same individual has come to terms with their altered functioning and lowered their expectations of their ideal self in line with this change in actual self. The gap has therefore diminished and QoL will have improved, even if it may not be back to the initial level. As health improves so expectations of self increase and QoL returns to its original set point.

One idea about how we arrive at this ideal and actual self is the social comparison theory. This theory proposes that we make QoL judgements by comparing ourselves, our status and/or our situation with that of others (Suls et al. 2002). Sometimes we choose to compare ourselves to others who are in a more fortunate situation than we are, at other times we might compare ourselves to individuals or groups who are worse off than we are. Either of these comparisons can result in enhancement or diminishment of our own situation – and therefore either widen or shrink the gap between reality and aspiration. For example, a patient undergoing NPWT might compare themselves with someone else who has undergone the same treatment for the same diagnosis and is now cured, and believe that they too will get better. The cured role model therefore provides hope and inspiration by demonstrating what can be achieved (Suls et al. 2002). Alternatively comparison to someone who is more fortunate could suggest to an individual that they are relatively disadvantaged, leading to a reduction in QoL assessment. In contrast a patient being treated with traditional wound care might look at someone who they see as worse off than they are (undergoing NPWT for example) and feel better about their own situation so enhancing their own perceived QoL, or remind them that their own status could also decline leading to reduced QoL. So just what influences whether or not social comparison serves a self-enhancement function?

One factor that may influence these social comparisons is affect (Wheeler and Miyake 1992). This is consistent with affect-cognition theories in psychology, which suggests that negative emotions elicit negative thoughts about the self and *vice versa*. Thus individuals who are feeling positive will further enhance these feelings by making a comparison that either re-enforces the superiority of their own position or provides inspiration and hope for the future; individuals who are feeling unhappy will boost their misery further by making unfavourable comparisons of their own situation to that of others or through the despair that is aroused by identification with those who are in a worse situation than themselves. This may also explain in part, the relationship between QoL – our cognitive assessment of our situation – and wellbeing – how positive we feel. Thus by compelling individuals into making favourable social comparisons, the presence of positive emotion may mediate (protect) against some of the more detrimental effects of living with a wound.

Measuring Quality of Life

HRQoL measurement has been considered one of the most difficult and challenging areas faced by health care professionals (Lyons 2005). This is in part due to the subjective nature of QoL, which means that it cannot be measured by objective observation, it can only be assessed by patient self-report measurement. Furthermore such patient reports cannot be verified by another individual, or by observation alone (Colver 2006).

HRQoL can be assessed using either qualitative or quantitative techniques; in practice quantitative fixed-response measures such as questionnaires are normally used in a clinical setting. Such quantitative HRQoL measurement usually takes one of two possible approaches, generic or condition specific assessment.

Generic questionnaires measure broad aspects of HRQoL and provide a general sense of the effects of health on wellbeing and function. Questions cover general issues of health such as whether or not an individual has experienced any aches or pains and what impact that has had on their QoL. The questions are therefore applicable to the general population and measures can be applied to any disease group and even healthy individuals.

The second approach uses measures that are specific to a condition or population. Questions therefore concern issues related to a particular illness and its treatment. Thus a measure designed to assess the HRQoL of a patient with a wound, would ask about the impact of wound related symptoms such as wound pain and exudate on an individual's QoL. Questions are also likely to address issues such as the effect of treatments factors such as dressings change, compression bandaging or NPWT. Thus a condition-specific measure covers issues pertaining to a specific disease or population and as such can only be applied to the disease or population for which they were developed

Because of this specificity, such instruments are likely to be more powerful at detecting intervention effects than generic instruments. This is not to say that condition–specific instruments provide "better" assessments of HRQoL, rather the choice of generic or specific depends on the purpose of the assessment. Thus generic measures should be used for comparisons of HRQoL across different wound types, and between those with a chronic wound and those without. They can therefore be administered to different populations to examine the impact of general health care initiatives and as such offer potential for measuring change in a population. Condition specific measures will however be more useful when making comparisons within a specific disease or population – for example when considering the relative benefits and costs of different treatment regimes for individuals with wounds. Examples of both generic and disease specific measures commonly applied to wound care populations is given in Table 4.1.

Whilst generic and disease specific measures have a different focus for their questions, both share a multidimensional construct that integrates a number of features including physical, social and psychological functioning (see Table 4.2).

TABLE 4.1 Measures of quality of life typically administered to patients with wounds

Measures of quality of life	Type
Cardiff wound impact schedule (CWIS)	Wound specific
Charing cross venous leg ulcer questionnaire (CCVLUQ)	Wound specific
Sheffield Preference-based Venous Ulcer questionnaire (SPVU-5D)	Wound specific
Skindex	Wound specific
Hyland New Ulcer Specific Tool	Wound specific
WoundQoL	Wound specific
Nottingham health profile (NHP)	Generic
Philadelphia geriatric centre multi-level assessment instrument	Generic
SF-36	Generic
EuroQoL (EQ-5D)	Generic

In practice, many measures follow the WHO statement that health is "a state of complete physical, mental, and social well-being; not merely the absence of disease" (WHO 1948) as their conceptual foundation and often focus specifically on the impact of illness and treatment on these aspects of daily life. According to Varni et al. (2003) HRQoL instruments must be multidimensional, consisting at the *minimum* of the physical, mental, and social health dimensions delineated by the World Health Organization (WHO 1948). These core components of physical, mental and social functioning may therefore be supplemented with additional dimensions such as patient satisfaction and spirituality (Cella 1997). Table 4.2 clearly demonstrates this. All three generic and three wound specific measures cover the minimum domains of physical, social and emotional functioning. However each measure also includes a range of other domains including vitality, cosmeis, pain and smell.

Table 4.2 Domains covered by quality of life typically administered to patients with wounds

SF36	EQ-5D	Nottingham health profile	Charing cross VLU	Cardiff wound profile	SPVU-5D
8 Domains:	5 Domains:	6 Domains:	4 Domains:	4 Domains:	5 Domains:
Physical functioning	Mobility	Physical mobility	Domestic activities	Physical symptoms	Mobility
Role limitations-physical	Self-care				
Bodily pain	Pain/discomfort	Pain			Pain
General health					
Energy & vitality		Energy			
Social functioning	Usual activities	Social isolation	Social interaction	Social life	Social activities
Role limitations – emotional	Anxiety/depression	Emotional reactions	Emotional status	Well-being	Mood

Measuring Quality of Life

Mental health | Sleep | Cosmesis | HRQoL | Smell

Both generic and wound specific measures of HRQoL which can be used with a wound population are therefore readily available. A recent review (Palfreyman et al. 2010) found that generic measures such as SF36, NHP and EQ-5D did demonstrate that individuals with wounds had reduced QoL in comparison to the general population. However the ability of measures such as CWIS and CCVLUQ to detect changes in QoL as patients healed was found to be limited. This is in part because the measures all include questions only relevant when an ulcer is present, limiting their applicability following healing. CWIS was also criticised for attempting to be too broad in its application. The CWIS was designed to be applied to all chronic wound types ranging from pressure ulcer, through sinuses, diabetes, trauma and leg ulcers. Unfortunately the significant differences in impact seen between these different types of wound seems to have seriously limited the sensitivity of this measure. This underlines the importance of specificity for increasing sensitivity to change and also underlines the importance of ensuring you choose the right tool when measuring HRQoL. For example Higginson and Carr (2001) suggest a two step method to choosing and implementing a QoL measure in a clinical setting. The first step (choosing the measure) advises clinicians to answer ten questions about the measures being reviewed including the relevance of the domains covered, the similarity of the population and setting in which the measure was developed to the one about to be assessed, the reliability and validity of the measure, length of time taken to complete, and easy of use. The second step – introducing the measure into practice is considered later in this chapter.

Measuring Well-Being

Increasing importance is being placed on the well-being of the individual living with a wound, as evidenced by the introduction of an International Consensus Document (2012) on well-being which has at its heart the aim of ensuring 'that

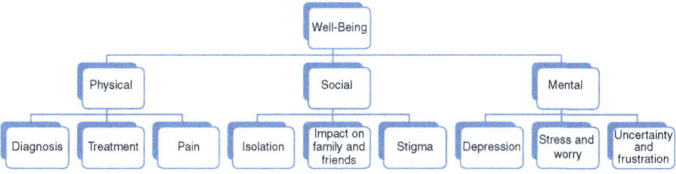

FIGURE 4.3 Domains of well-being proposed by International Consensus Document 2012

wellbeing is the principle focus of care' (International Consensus 2012). However, whilst this document provides an excellent starting point for taking this vital work forward, there remains much to be done in relation to defining dimensions and developing assessment tools. For example, whilst the consensus document tries to make a differentiation between QoL and well-being, the domains of well-being described appear to be identical to those used traditionally used in QoL definitions (physical, mental and social well-being) with the addition of spiritual and cultural well-being (see Fig. 4.3) The distinction between QoL as a cognitive appraisal and well-being as an emotional response appears to be missing.

As already described, we can see QoL and well-being as distinct yet related concepts. Both are influenced by a patient's context – the wounds, its symptoms, treatment, changes in social and physical functioning (e.g. pain). In addition each influences the other in a continual feedback loop. Thus it would be possible for a patient to be caught in a downward spiral where increasing pain reduces QoL and well-being, resulting in reduced social contacts, in turn leading to further reductions in QoL and well-being (see Fig. 4.4). It can be hypothesised that by making a break in this cycle, potentially by boosting a patient's psychological resources (improving coping, or social support for example) well-being can be enhanced and patient outcomes can be improved (Upton et al. 2014).

Furthermore, in contrast to the many measures of HRQoL available for use in wound care, there are currently no

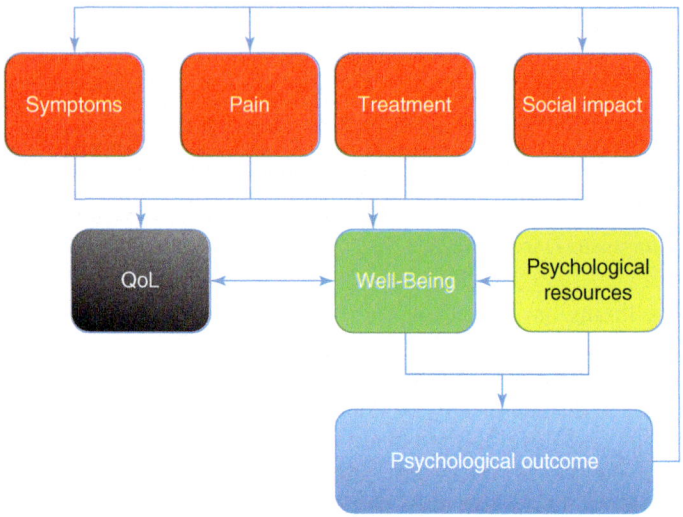

Figure 4.4 A hypothesised model of wellbeing

appropriate measures of patient well-being. Whilst the CWIS (Price and Harding 2004) does include a well-being scale, the scale is limited by its focus on questions concerning negative affect such as anxiety and worry. It seems therefore that there is a gap in the assessment process, since QoL and well-being represent quite different aspects of the patient experience.

As it has developed, HRQoL has evolved into a measure of deficit of daily living. Thus HRQoL tools typically ask patients to consider whether their health problem hinders physical functioning (e.g. getting dressed), disrupts social activities (e.g. seeing friends), prevents productivity behaviours (e.g. going to work), or causes emotional problems such as depression, anxiety or stress. Whilst it is of course vital that any restrictions of physical, social and mental functioning are documented, focusing solely on these aspects of the patient experience is rather limited, especially since it emphasises the deficits in a patient's standard of living. It is also important that an absence of negative affect is not take as an indicator of positive mental health; just because a patient is not depressed, this does not mean they have hope or happiness. Likewise, if a patient is anxious or worried, it should not be assumed that they therefore are unhappy or feel socially isolated. It is perfectly possible – indeed likely – that a patient will experience a complex mixture of positive and negative affect, just as we all do everyday. Indeed, some studies have shown that patients may experience conflicting emotions – for example feeling both hopeful and pessimistic or despairing about the future (Ebbeskog and Ekman 2001a; Hopkins 2004a).

Which brings us to the second problem of not assessing well-being, which is that not doing so ignores the potential psychological resources which an individual may (or may not) have at their disposal; resources such as hope, self-efficacy and adaptive coping which make patients more resilient when present, and especially vulnerable when absent. Identifying and working to improve reduced well-being should be one of the goals of clinical care. Indeed, the potentially protective value of well-being should not be dismissed lightly, given the known link between psychological health and physical healing (Upton and Solowiej 2010). Thus it is essential that clinicians consider both the cognitive and emotional responses of a patient to their wound.

Factors Which Impact on Quality of Life and Well-Being

The evidence suggests that the QoL of patients with wounds is compromised in the three primary domains – physical, psychological and social. Several factors contribute to this reduced QoL, with the most obvious being the physical symptoms which patients experience. Pain has been found to be a significant issue (Walshe 1995; see Chap. 2), and may relate to either wound pain or the pain related to dressing change (Langemo 2005). Sleep disturbance (Byrne and Kelly 2010; Upton and Andrews 2013), and problems with mobility are also likely to reduce physical functioning and limit daily activities (Persoon et al 2004). Lack of energy, which also limits physical functioning, has also been reported in some studies (Fagervik-Morton and Price 2009).

Psychological functioning is also reduced in people with wounds, with one of the most commonly reported responses being depression or feeling 'low' (e.g. Finlayson et al. 2010; Finlayson et al. 2011; Jones et al. 2006; Jones et al. 2008a; Byrne and Kelly 2010; Upton et al. 2012); some people even report feeling so low that they have thoughts of suicide (Byrne and Kelly 2010; Mapplebeck 2008). Physical symptoms such as pain and length of healing time have been linked with feelings of depression (Byrne and Kelly 2010). Other factors which have been shown to increase problems of mood include limited knowledge of one's condition and treatment (Douglas 2001; Flaherty 2005); a lack of confidence in healthcare professionals (Mudge et al. 2006); being cared for by unfamiliar nurses (Hopkins 2004a; Byrne and Kelly 2010; Walshe 1995; Brown 2005a, b); feeling ignored or mistreated by clinicians (Ebbeskog and Emami 2005); and finally, conflicts in the nurse-patient relationship due to a difference in focus on treatment outcomes versus symptom-relief (Brown 2005a, b).

In addition to low mood, studies have highlighted feelings of embarrassment, anxiety and reduced self-confidence in relation to body image; more extreme emotional responses to body image such as shame, disgust and self-loathing have also been recorded (Hopkins 2004a; Byrne and Kelly 2010; Jones et al. 2008a; Mapplebeck 2008; Douglas 2001; Ebbeskog and Ekman 2001a; Mudge et al. 2006; Flaherty 2005). Fear of amputation may also be an issue for people with venous leg ulcers (Mapplebeck 2008; Hopkins 2004a). Other high arousal feelings such as anger and frustration have also been noted (Jones et al. 2008a; Mapplebeck 2008). Finally, patients may report feeling helpless, as though they lack control (Walshe 1995; Jones et al. 2008a).

Social functioning has also been found to be compromised in people with chronic wounds (Adni et al. 2012; see Chap. 1). Problems associated with having a wound (in particular exudate and odour) may lead to social isolation (Herber et al. 2007; Price 2009), social withdrawal (Fagervik-Morton and Price 2009) and changes in relationships with others, particularly carers Fagervik-Morton and Price 2009). Treatment type may also prohibit involvement in social activities (Upton et al. 2013). All of this may lead to loneliness (Green and Jester 2009) as well as increasing psychological distress and other negative emotional responses. In addition to this some studies have noted a relationship between reduced capacity to work, limitations of social functioning and financial difficulties (Green and Jester 2009).

In contrast to what we know about changes in QoL for patients with wounds, little is known about changes in well-being. To date a small number of studies have demonstrated the positive emotions that some people with VLU experience despite living with a range of negative consequences (Hopkins 2004a; Flett et al. 1994). Research into other chronic health conditions suggests that such positivity in the face of adversity can be explained by mediating variables such as coping style, personality, hope, and resilience (Stanton et al. 2001). Certainly hope and resilience have also been reported in VLU patients (Hopkins 2004a; Ebbeskog and Ekman 2001a; Byrne and Kelly 2010) and it has been proposed that these are protective variables that must be explored further in relation to well-being in wounds (Upton et al. 2014).

Implications for Clinical Practice

Studies reviewed in this chapter have highlighted a number of issues that directly impact upon the QoL and well-being of patients with wounds and which have implications for clinical practice including the importance of ensuring:

- Effective assessment and management of pain and stress;
- Effective strategies to manage wound exudate and malodour;

- Information sharing with patients and carers'
- Comprehensive care pathways that include assessment of QoL and well-being;
- Clinician and patient relationships are based on collaboration

Taking a patient centred approach to wound management should help ensure that these concerns are addressed (Reddy et al. 2003). It has been suggested that patients' greatest problems occur because clinicians do not hear (or understand) what they are saying in the context of their lives (Husband 2001). For example, Jones et al. (2002) discovered that the emotional distress presented by patients often goes undetected by clinicians and carers.

During clinical assessment, it is therefore essential that patients' views and opinions are heard. One way of ensuring this is for clinicians to use terminology that patients can understand (Eagle 2009). Using this model, a patient's perceived needs in relation to their wound management can be taken into account; for example, wound healing may not be their top priority, but rather freedom from exudate or pain relief. The emphasis is therefore on information and knowledge provision, and collaborative decision making between patient and clinician. Such collaboration in treatment and management decisions fosters self-control whilst empowering patients. Indeed, the patient-clinician relationship is a vital part of the treatment planning process (Eagle 2009).

Assessing patient QoL and well-being is also an important part of developing a treatment plan, and provides an effective way of giving the patient a voice. Furthermore, assessing the psychosocial factors associated with living with a wound should be a routine part of practice, since factors such as pain and stress can impact on healing and ulcer recurrence (Moffatt et al. 2008; Cole-King and Harding 2001; Woo 2010; Upton and Solowiej 2010; see Chap. 3). This delayed healing can result either from the direct impact of psychological difficulties on physiological healing processes, or indirectly, as a result of patients not adhering to treatment (Finlayson et al. 2010). Routine assessment of QoL provides access to

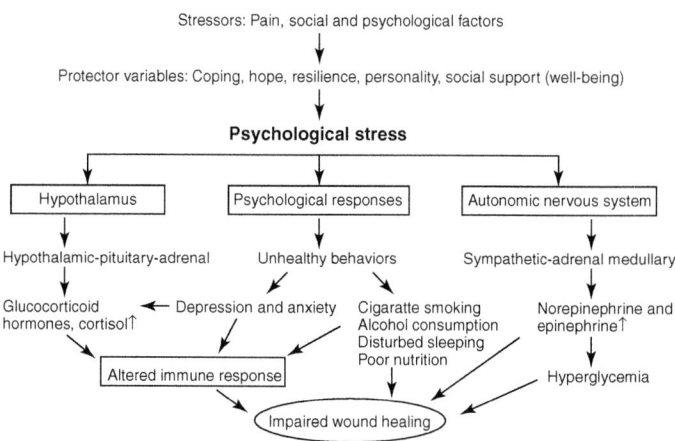

FIGURE 4.5 The importance of wellbeing for physical and mental health

these psychosocial factors and allows clinician to put interventions in place to address any deficits in functioning such as stress or depression.

In the same way assessing well-being is also important, as the presence of positive psychological factors associated with well-being – such as hope and optimism – are likely to enable better overall psychological health, increased treatment concordance, and improved healing speed. Such an association has been discovered in other long term conditions, with positive well-being being related to improved outcomes (Rozanski et al. 1999).

Whilst it is currently unclear why some people with wounds are able to retain a sense of positivity and well-being in spite of their difficulties, insights derived from other conditions strengthen the view that it is not the wound per se that is the decisive factor in wellbeing, but rather that fundamental psychosocial factors are protective (Rozanski et al. 1999). Identification of these factors is important so that maladaptive elements can be replaced with protective ones. Figure 4.5 demonstrates a possible mechanism through which wellbeing may protect against psychological stressors which impact on wound healing.

Clinicians are also likely to have an important role in influencing patient well-being and the subsequent healing process; for example, treatment factors such as patient knowledge and the quality of the therapeutic relationship are known to affect how patients feel (Douglas 2001; Hopkins 2004a). Whilst these issues still need to be explored further, it is important for healthcare professionals to be aware of the indirect impact that they may have on patient well-being.

Most importantly, clinicians need to be aware of the significance of assessing and monitoring well-being. Knowing whether a patient feels positive about themselves and the future is important for factors such as mental health and treatment concordance. The current emphasis on QoL does not allow such insight and a shift in focus is needed. Clinicians and researchers must move away from solely assessing QoL – deficits of daily living – and towards exploring individual well-being – the presence of positive emotions and hope for the future. As research in this area evolves, and suitable evaluation tools and guidelines are produced, clinicians working with people with wounds will need to develop their assessment approach accordingly. Furthermore, a move from the reactive to the proactive; a recognition of the importance of the patient experience of having a wound- their emotional reactions, hopes and expectations – will enable health care professionals to better support patients to cultivate positive psychological resources. This will result in improved patient adherence, better healing rates, reduced treatment costs and, ultimately, a better overall patient outcome.

Conclusion

This chapter has demonstrated that QoL and well-being are related, but distinct concepts: QoL refers to a cognitive appraisal of our health status, whereas well-being is the emotional response. We have seen that patient QoL can be significantly altered by the presence of a wound and that this in turn can impair healing. In contrast, patient well-being appears to provide a protective mechanism, through which it might be possible to promote physical and mental health. In practice, clinicians should pay attention to patient's QoL and well-being as a mechanism for giving the patient a voice, and an input to their care plan, as this assessment shifts the focus from the wound and physical outcomes such as healing, to the whole person, with the aim of making living with a wound the best it can be.

References

Adni T, Martin K, Mudge E. The psychosocial impact of chronic wounds on patients with severe epidermolysis bullosa. J Wound Care. 2012;21(11):528–38.

Brown A. Chronic leg ulcers, part 1: do they affect a patient's social life? Br J Nurs. 2005a;14(17):894–8.

Brown A. Chronic leg ulcers, part 2: do they affect a patient's social life? Br J Nurs. 2005b;14(18):986–9.

Brown G. Speech to the volunteering conference, London, 2005c. 31 Jan 2005.

Byrne O, Kelly M. Living with a chronic leg ulcer. J Commun Nurs. 2010;24(5):46–54.

Cella DF. FACIT Manual. Manual of the functional assessment of chronic illness therapy (FACIT) measurement system. Version 4; 1997

Centers for Disease Control and Prevention. Well-being concepts. 2011. Available from: http://www.cdc.gov/hrqol/wellbeing.htm.

Cole-King A, Harding KG. Psychological factors and delayed healing in chronic wounds. Psychosom Med. 2001;63:216–20.

Colver A. Study protocol: SPARCLE–a multi-centre European study of the relationship of environment to participation and quality of life in children with cerebral palsy. BMC Public Health. 2006;6(1):105.

Douglas V. Living with a chronic leg ulcer: an insight into patients' experiences and feelings. J Wound Care. 2001;10(9):355–60.

Draper P, Thompson DR. The quality of life- a concept for research practice. J Res Nurs. 2001;6(3):648–57.

Eagle M. Wound assessment: the patient and the wound. Wound Essentials. 2009;4:14–24.

Ebbeskog B, Ekman S-L. Elderly persons' experiences of living with venous leg ulcer: living in a dialectical relationship between freedom and imprisonment. Scand J Caring Sci. 2001a;15:235–43.

Ebbeskog B, Ekman S-L. Older patients' experience of dressing changes on venous leg ulcers: more than just a docile patient. J Clin Nurs. 2001b;14(10):1223–31.

Ebbeskog B, Emami A. Older patients' experience of dressing changes on venous leg ulcers: more than just a docile patient. J Clin Nurs. 2005;14(10):1223–31.

Eiser C, Eiser J. Social comparisons and quality of life among survivors of childhood cancer and their mothers. Psychol Health. 2000; 15:435–50.

Fagervik-Morton H, Price P. Chronic ulcers and everyday living: patients' perspective in the United Kingdom. Wounds. 2009;21(12):318–23.

Fayers P, Machin D. Quality of life: the assessment, analysis and interpretation of patient-reported outcomes. Chichester: John Wiley & Sons Ltd; 2007.

Finlayson K, Edwards H, Courtney M. The impact of psychosocial factors on adherence to compression therapy to prevent recurrence of venous leg ulcers. J Clin Nurs. 2010;29:1289–97.

Finlayson K, Edwards H, Courtney M. Relationships between preventive activities, psychosocial factors and recurrence of venous leg ulcers: a prospective study. J Adv Nurs. 2011;67(10):2180–90.

Flaherty E. The views of patients living with healed venous leg ulcers. Nurs Stand. 2005;19(45):78–89.

Flett R, Harcourt B, Alpass F. Psychosocial aspects of chronic lower leg ulceration in the elderly. West J Nurs Res. 1994;16(2): 183–93.

Galloway S, Bell D, Hamilton C, Scullion AC. Well-being and quality of life: measuring the benefits of culture and sport- a literature review and thinkpiece. Series: Education (Scotland. Social Research), Edinburgh: Scottish Government; 2006.

Green J, Jester R. Health-related quality of life and chronic venous leg ulceration: part 1. Wound Care. 2009;14(12):12–7.

Herber OR, Schnepp W, Rieger MA. A systematic review on the impact of leg ulceration on patients' quality of life. Health Qual Life Outcomes. 2007;5(44):1–12.

Higginson IJ, Carr AJ. Using quality of life measures in the clinical setting. BMJ. 2001;1294:322–30.

Hopkins A. Disrupted lives: investigating coping strategies for non-healing leg ulcers. Br J Nurs. 2004a;13(9):556–63.

Hopkins A. The use of qualitative research methodologies to explore leg ulceration. J Tissue Viability. 2004b;14(4):142–7.

Husband LL. Venous ulceration: the pattern of pain and the paradox. Clin Effect Nurs. 2001;5(1):35–40.

International consensus. Optimising wellbeing in people living with a wound. An expert working group review. London: Wounds International; 2012. Available from: http://www.woundsinternational.com.

Jones A, Spindler H, Jorgensen MM, Zachariae R. The effect of situation-evoked anxiety and gender on pain report using the cold pressor test. Scand J Psychol. 2002;43(4):307–13.

Jones J, Barr W, Robinson J, Carlisle C. Depression in patients with chronic venous ulceration. Br J Nurs. 2006;15(11):17–23.

Jones JE, Robinson J, Barr W, Carlisle C. Impact of exudate and odour from chronic venous leg ulceration. Nurs Stand. 2008a; 22(45):53–61.

Jones RA, Taylor AG, Bourguignon C. Family interactions among African American Prostate Cancer Survivors. Fam Community Health. 2008b;31(3):213–20.

Lach LM, Ronen GM, Rosenbaum PL, Cunningham C, Boyle MH, Bowman S, Streiner D. Health-related quality of life in youth with epilepsy: theoretical model for clinicians and researchers. Part I: the role of epilepsy and co-morbidity. Qual Life Res. 2006;15(7): 1161–71.

Langemo DK. Quality of life and pressure ulcers: what is the impact? Wounds. 2005;17(1):3–7.

Lyons G. The life satisfaction matrix: an instrument and procedure for assessing the subjective quality of life of individuals with profound multiple disabilities. J Intellect Disabil Res. 2005;49(10): 766–9.

Mapplebeck L. Case study: psychosocial aspects of chronic bilateral venous leg ulcers. Br J Community Nurs. 2008;13(3):S33–8.

Moffatt C, Vowden K, Price P, Vowden P. Psychosocial factors in delayed healing. In hard-to-heal wounds: a holistic approach. European Wound Management Association Position Statement. 2008. Available from: http://ewma.org/fileadmin/user_upload/EWMA/pdf/Position_Documents/2008/English_EWMA_Hard2Heal_2008.pdf.

Morrison RS, Meier DE, Capello CF. Geriatric palliative care. New York: Oxford University Press; 2003.

Mudge E, Holloway S, Simmonds W, Price P. Living with venous leg ulceration: issues concerning adherence. Br J Nurs. 2006;15(21): 1166–71.

Palfreyman SM, Tod AM, Brazier JE, Michaels JA. A systematic review of health-related quality of life instruments used for people with venous ulcers: an assessment of their suitability and psychometric properties. J Clin Nurs. 2010;19(19):2673–703.

Pawlyn J, Carnaby S. Profound intellectual and multiple disabilities: nursing complex needs. Chichester: Wiley-Blackwell; 2009.

Persoon A, Heinen M, van der Vleuten C, de Rooij M, van de Kerkhof P, van Achterberg T. Leg ulcers: a review of their impact on daily life. J Clin Nurs. 2004;13(3):341–54.

Price P, Harding KG. Cardiff wound impact schedule: the development of a condition-specific questionnaire to assess health related quality of life in patients with chronic wounds of the lower limb. Int Wound J. 2004;1(1):10–3.

Rapley M. Quality of life research: a critical introduction. London: Sage; 2003.

Reddy M, Kohr R, Queen D, Keast D, Sibbald RG. Practical treatment of wound pain and trauma: a patient-centered approach. An overview. Ostomy Wound Manage. 2003;49(4 Suppl):2–15.

Rozanski A, Blumenthanl JA, Kaplan J. Impact of psychological factors on the pathogenesis of cardiovascular disease and implications for therapy. Circulation. 1999;99:2192–217.

Sen CK, Gordillo GM, Roy S, Kirsner R, Lambert L, Hunt TK, Longaker MT. Human skin wounds: a major and snowballing threat to public health and the economy. Wound Repair Regen. 2009;17(6):763–71.

Shukla VK, Shukla D, Singh A, Tripathi AK, Sushil J, Somprakas B. Risk assessment for pressure ulcer: a hospital-based study. J Wound Ostomy Cont Nurs. 2008;35(4):407–11.

Stanton AL, Collins CA, Sworowski L. Adjustment to chronic illness: theory and research. In: Baum A, Revenson TA, Singer JE, editors. Handbook of health psychology. Mahwah: Lawrence Erlbaum Associate; 2001. p. 387–404.

Suls J, Martin R, Wheeler L. Social comparison: why, with whom, and with what effect? J Assoc Psychol Sci. 2002;11(5):159–63.

Upton D, Andrews A. Sleep disruption in patients with chronic leg ulcers. J Wound Care. 2013;22(8):389–94.

Upton D, Andrews A. Negative pressure wound therapy: improving the patient experience, part two of three. J Wound Care. 2013a;22(11):582–91.

Upton D, Andrews A. Negative pressure wound therapy: improving the patient experience, part one of three. J Wound Care. 2013b;22(10):552–7.

Upton D, Andrews A. Pain and trauma in negative pressure wound therapy: a review. Int Wound J. 2013; Advance online publication.

Upton D, Solowiej K. Pain and stress as contributors to delayed wound healing. Wound Pract Res. 2010;18(3):114–22.

Upton D, Hender C, Solowiej K. Mood disorders in patients with acute and chronic wounds: a health professional perspective. J Wound Care. 2012;21(1):42–8.

Upton D, Stephens D, Andrews A. Patients' experience of negative pressure wound therapy. J Wound Care. 2013;22(1):34–9.

Upton D, Andrews A, Upton P. Venous leg ulcers: what about well-being? J Wound Care. 2014;23(1):14–7.

Varni JW, Burwinkle TM, Seid M, Skarr D. The PedsQL™ 4.0 as a pediatric population health measure: feasibility, reliability, and validity. Ambul Pediatr. 2003;3:329–41.

Wallander JL. Quality of life measurement in children and adolescents: Issues, instruments, and applications. J Clin Psychol. 2001;57(4):571–85.

Walshe C. Living with a venous leg ulcer: a descriptive study of patients' experiences. J Adv Nurs. 1995;22(6):1092–100.

Wheeler L, Miyake K. Social comparison in every day life. J Pers Soc Psychol. 1992;62(5):760–73.

WHO. Preamble to the constitution of the world health organization as adopted by the international health conference, New York, 19–22 June, 1946; signed on 22 July 1946 by the representatives of 61 States (Official Records of the World Health Organization, no. 2, p. 100) and entered into force on 7 April 1948; 1948.

WHO. WHOQOL: measuring quality of life. Geneva: WHO; 1997.

Woo KY. Wound-related pain: anxiety, stress and wound healing. Wounds UK. 2010;6(4):92–8.

Zikmund V. Health, well-being, and the quality of life: Some psychosomatic reflections. Neuro Endocrinol Lett. 2003;24(6):401.

Chapter 5
Different Wound Type

> Box 5.1: Key Points
> - Wounds and wound care have a significant psychosocial components and it is important that these are recognised, appreciated and managed.
> - Although there are many commonalities there are also subtle differences of the psychological concomitants of different wound types and this chapter outlines some of these.
> - Burns are a traumatic wound type that has significant psychological consequences for the individual patient, some of which may be related to pre-existing psychological morbidity.
> - Psychological issues are significant consequences for those with diabetic foot issues that may result in further ulceration- psychotherapeutic interventions can reduce psychological distress and prevent further physical deterioration.
> - Pressure Ulcers can have a significant impact on quality of life and of key importance in this can be the nurse-patient relationship.
> - Venous Leg Ulcers are a common condition, which can be extremely painful: better social support can have a positive impact on the pain experienced.

Summary

Although there are many commonalities in the lived experience of those with different forms of wounds, there are also important differences. This chapter highlights some of these differences but, in addition, uses the different forms of wounds to highlight the importance of psychological variables in wounds and wound care. For example, for those with traumatic burn injuries it is important to understand any underlying pre-existing psychological morbidity. This is outlined in this chapter, along with some potential methods for assessing these. For those with diabetic foot ulcers, the potential impact of psychological distress on further ulceration is outlined along with some methods for ameliorating this. Pressure ulcers, a significant condition that impacts on many, can have serious implications on health related quality of life and factors associated with this- in particular the nurse-patient relationship- are outlined and explained. Finally, the pain associated with Venous Leg Ulcers is outlined and the potential importance of both assessment- through the verbal descriptions associated with pain- and social interventions are emphasised. Overall, this chapter highlights the importance of a psychological understanding in a range of wound types.

Introduction

This chapter will serve to illustrate some of the key issues (e.g. pain, well-being, communication) raised in other chapters by applying them to different wound types. There are a number of different wounds that health care professionals may encounter and each of these may have their own specifically related psychological factors. For example, there may be different psychological consequences dependent on whether the individual has a traumatic wound, including surgical or burn related, a diabetic foot ulcer, a pressure ulcer, or venous or arterial leg ulcers. These wounds each have their own complexities and important differences exist between them.

Not only can they differ in relation to their physiology and their clinical care, but they can also have substantial differences in the psychological impact on patients. Hence, it is not only important for health professionals to acknowledge and understand such difference, it is also important that they incorporate such knowledge within their daily wound-care regimes (see Box 5.1). This will be the focus of this particular chapter- exploring the psychological concomitants of a variety of different wound types and the impact that this has on individual care.

Burns

Trauma wounds are often accompanied by serious psychological implications, severely disrupting normal daily activities (Coker et al. 2008). One of the most severe traumas a person can endure is that of a burn injury (Klinge et al. 2009; Hodder et al. 2014). Sustaining a burn injury can cause both significant psychological distress and physical pain. For example, fire-related trauma wounds can result in a number of negative medical consequences, including hypovolemic shock, sepsis, multi-organ failure and, subsequently, mortality (Young 2002; Herndon 2007). Psychosocial difficulties associated with a burn injury can include: financial strain, relationship difficulties, loss of physical functions, emotional dysfunction, disfigurement and body image concerns (Hodder et al. 2014; Esselman et al. 2006; Partridge and Robinson 1995).

Mortality rate associated with major burns has decreased dramatically over the last 50 years. This can be attributed to a number of factors, whether it being the advanced knowledge surrounding the pathophysiology of burn injury (Young 2002; Herndon 2007), or the establishment of a number of specialised burn units (Diver 2008) and advancements in wound care (White and Renz 2008). As a result, multi-disciplinary teams have been developed which focus not only on the surgical, medical and reconstructive stages of burns treatment, but also on the psychological and psychosocial well-being of burn patients (Young 2002; Herndon 2007). Hence, as mortality has decreased, the importance placed upon the psychological well-being of burn survivors has increased substantially (Klinge et al. 2009; Smith et al. 2006).

During the first year following a burn trauma, a patient is highly vulnerable being susceptible to experiences of anxiety, depression, psychosis and delirium (Edwards et al. 2007). Indeed, studies have suggested that psychological recovery parallels physical recovery (Smith et al. 2006). Studies have highlighted the predominance of anxiety and depression to be reported as long-term symptoms (Edwards et al. 2007), with the prevalence rate of overall psychological consequences being between 10 and 65 % (Edwards et al. 2007; De Young et al. 2012; van Loey et al. 2012). Personality type, coping styles and situational factors have been found to be associated with post-burn psychological adjustment (Herndon 2007; van Loey et al. 2012). Park et al. (2008) discovered that combined with the previous risk factors, employment, marital status, financial position, and social support can predict psychological adjustment and psychosocial outcomes of burn patients. Similarly, van Loey et al. (2012) reported that quality of life in the long-term was influenced by physical recovery, number of surgical interventions and psychological disorder (particularly posttraumatic stress disorder). Hence, it is essential for clinicians to identify potential risk factors than may impede the psychological adjustment of wound patients. Klinge et al. (2009), in their review of the burn wounds literature, highlighted six factors that may place a role in the adjustment of post-burn patients;

1. Psychological status pre-burn;
2. Vocational status pre-burn;
3. Coping style and personality type;
4. Social support and network;
5. Burn characteristics;
6. Gender.

An interesting point to note is that the authors reported that burn patients had a higher incidence of pre-existing psychopathology when compared with the general population. This has been highlighted previously by findings that pre-existing psychological disorders, substance and alcohol abuse and depression have a causal role in the aetiology of the burn itself (Dyster-Aas et al. 2008). Hence, it has been suggested that patients who have sustained a burn wound may have had diminished cognitive processes related to such pre-burn factors that, in turn, predisposed them to such an injury (Klinge et al. 2009). For example, a meta-analysis conducted by Noronha and Faust (2006) highlighted such a link with pre-existing psychopathology increasing post-burn psychological maladjustment.

Clinicians need to account for such issues within their daily wound care regimes as these psychological factors can have significant implications on satisfactory healing. For example, in a longitudinal study considering the relationship between pre-existing psychological issues and post-burn outcomes, the degree of impairment and healing rate of patient's experiencing differing levels of physical and psychological burden were examined (Fauerbach et al. 2005). It was found that an intervention based around the reduction of in-hospital distress and support psychological well-being proved to be as effective as surgical interventions. Research has heighted two forms of distress that burn patients' perceive during their hospital stay; alienation and anxiety (Fauerbach et al. 2007). Hence, clinicians need to be aware of these and the potential implications such psychological issues may have on the patient's subsequent experiences of pain, and further psychological distress. A cyclical relationship has been reported in patients with burn injuries, whereby depression and anxiety influences pain perception and reduced physical functioning which, in turn, further impacts anxiety and depression (Edwards et al. 2007). Hence, it is essential for clinicians to acknowledge and manage not only physical symptoms but emotional symptoms also (see Fig. 5.1). Such concurrent management strategies will then result in an improvement in a variety of long-term post-burn outcomes (including wound healing and physical functioning).

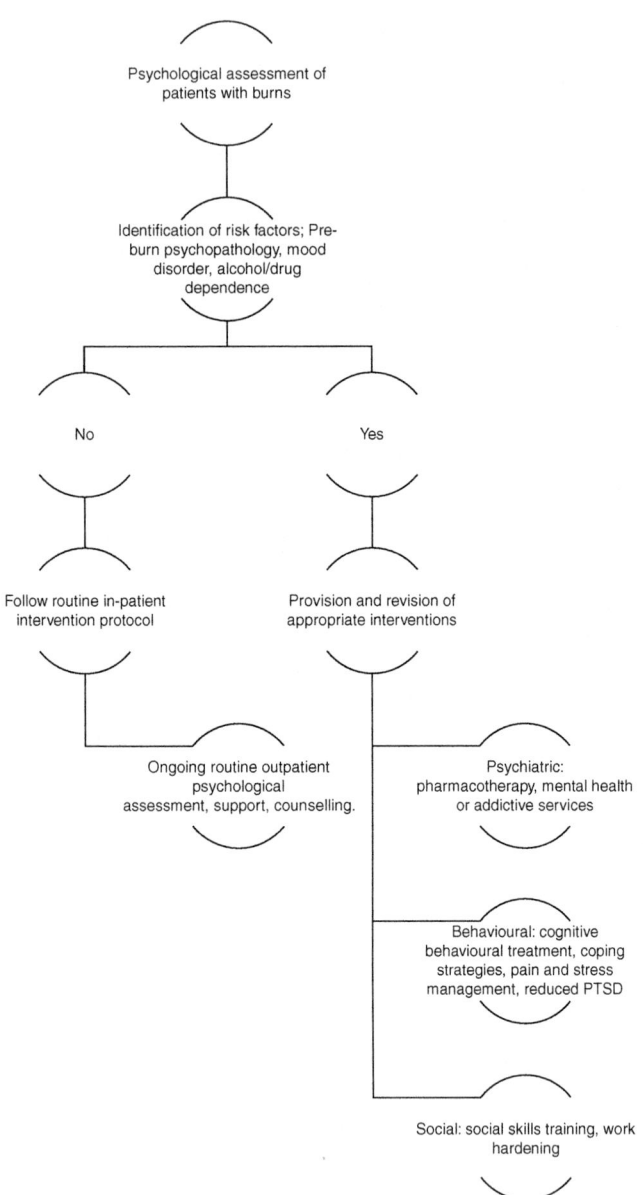

FIGURE 5.1 Proposed model of care: physical assessment after burn injury (Reproduced with permission from Klinge et al. (2009))

A large proportion of the burns literature also focusses on the relationship between personality type, coping strategies and post-burn adjustment. It has been reported that neuroticism, a trait largely associated with pessimism, negative affect and introversion, is one particular personality trait associated with adjustment difficulties (Klinge et al. 2009). Hence, it has been suggested that wound care clinicians need to integrate assessments that explore personality traits that may result in maladjustment and the adoption of dysfunctional coping strategies (Gilboa et al. 1999a, b). For example, patients who display optimism, 'self-mastery', or self-efficacy (ability to influence their outcomes) and hope prove to adjust more positively, whereas neurotic and introverted traits resulted in greater adjustment issues (Gilboa et al. 1999a, b).

Additionally, such patients were also more susceptible to post-traumatic stress disorder (PTSD; Fauerback et al. 1997; van Loey et al. 2003). Research has highlighted the prevalence of PTSD in burn survivors with van Loey et al. 2003 discovering 28 % of their participants to be meeting the DSM-IV criteria for either PTSD or partial PTSD. Furthermore, Bryant (1996) found that 60 % of burn patients were classified with PTSD or a subclinical form of PTSD. A major predictor of PTSD was the patient's concern about self-image related to the scarring resulting from the burn in addition to the adoption of avoidant coping styles (something that will be discussed later in relation to implications on wound healing). Hence, it is important for clinicians to acknowledge the associated between patients expressed concern over scarring and potential negative emotional reactions and adjustments.

Overall, it is essential that the patient who has suffered a wound is assessed adequately from a psychological perspective. There are a number of measures that may be useful in this regard. Table 5.1 highlights some of these and their benefits.

The measures reported in Table 5.1 are but some of the many measures that are available to the practising clinician to measure appropriate psychological variables. More of these are reported in other chapters, including the Chaps. 2, 3 and 7.

TABLE 5.1 Psychological assessment tools

Assessment tool	Comment
Stanford Acute Stress Reaction Questionnaire (SASQR): Cardena et al. (2000)	The SASQR is a 30-item instrument with various subscales and three additional questions relevant to the diagnosis of acute stress disorder, including a description of the event, how disturbing it was, and how many days the individual experienced the worst symptoms.
Alcohol misuse questionnaire scale (CAGE): Ewing (1984)	The CAGE questionnaire is a brief 4-item screening tool to identify alcohol misuse.
Beck depression inventory (BDI): Beck et al. (1961)	The BDI is a 21-item; self-report rating inventory that measures characteristic attitudes and symptoms of depression.
Body Esteem scale for adolescents and adults: Mendelson et al. (2001)	The scale consists of 21 items which evaluate the degree to which the individual attributes positive outcomes from their appearance.
Brief symptom inventory (BSI): Derogatis and Melisaratos (1983)	The BSI is a 53-item self-report inventory in which participant's rate the extent to which they have been bothered in the past week by various symptoms. The BSI has nine subscales designed to assess individual symptom groups: Somatization, obsessive-compulsive, interpersonal sensitivity, depression, anxiety, hostility, phobic anxiety, paranoid ideation and psychoticism. The BSI also includes three scales that capture global psychological distress
Impact of Event Scale- Revised (IES- R): Weiss and Marmar (1997)	A 15 item self-report scale assessing frequency of intrusive and avoidant phenomena associated with an event

TABLE 5.1 (continued)

Assessment tool	Comment
Burn Specific Anxiety Scale (BSPAS): Taal and Faber (1997)	The burn specific pain anxiety scale (BSPAS) is a nine-item self-report scale for the assessment of pain-related and anticipatory anxiety in burned patients.
Burn specific health scale (BSHS-A): Munster et al. (1987)	BSHS-A has 80 items across four domains (physical, mental, social, and general) and eight subscales (mobility and self-care, hand function, role activities, body image, affective, family/friends, sexual activity, and general health concerns).
Burn specific health scale revised (BSHS-R): Blalock et al. (1994)	BSHS-R is a revised version of the BSHR-A and has 31 items with two domains (physical and psychological) and seven sub-domains, and the BSHS-B has 40 items covering nine domains (heat sensitivity, affect, hand function, treatment regimen, work, sexuality, interpersonal relationships, simple abilities and body image).
Burn specific health scale (Brief) (BSHS-B): Kildal et al. (2001)	BSHS-B is a brief version it was developed because of perceived shortcomings with the other two versions in coverage of aspects of burn-specific health and inter-correlation of domains and sub-domains. The BSHS-B revealed three broad domains: affect and relations, function, and skin involvement.
Coping with burns questionnaire (CBQ): Willebrand et al. (2001)	The CBQ contains six factors corresponding to dimensions of coping: Revaluation/adjustment, Avoidance, Emotional support, Optimism/ problem solving, Self-control and Instrumental action.
Chronic stress scale (CSS): Norris et al. (1993)	A self-report survey that measures stress in seven life domains during the preceding 6 months.

(continued)

TABLE 5.1 (continued)

Assessment tool	Comment
COPE: Carver et al. (1989)	Assesses 13 lower-order strategies using four questions assigned to each of the following sub-scales: active coping, planning, suppression of competing activities, restraint coping, seeking social support for instrumental reasons, seeking social support for emotional reasons, positive reinterpretation and growth, acceptance, turning to religion, focus on and venting of emotions, denial, behavioural disengagement, and mental disengagement.
Brief COPE: Carver (1997)	A shortened version of the COPE designed for use when participant response burden is a considering factor. This questionnaire asks 28 questions on a four-point Likert scale.
NEO personality inventory: Costa and McCrae (1985)	A 300-question personality diagnostic measuring an individual's "Extraversion, Agreeableness, Conscientiousness, Neuroticism, and Openness to Experience.
NEO five-factor inventory (NEO-FFI) model: Costa and McCrae (1989)	The NEO-FFI is a 60 items using 5-point ratings: Openness, Conscientiousness, Extraversion, Agreeableness and Neuroticism.
Penn inventory (PENN) (PTSD tool): Hammarberg (1992)	The Penn Inventory is a 26-item self-report measure that assesses DSM-IV symptoms of Posttraumatic stress disorder. It can be used with clients with multiple traumatic experiences because symptoms are not keyed to any particular traumatic event.
Post-traumatic stress disorder symptom scale (PSS): Foa et al. (1993)	The PSS is a 17-item self-report measure of Post-traumatic stress disorder.

TABLE 5.1 (continued)

Assessment tool	Comment
Hospital anxiety and depression scale (HADS): Zigmond and Snaith (1983)	A brief assessment of anxiety and depression. It is a 14 item scale divided into 2 sub-scales for anxiety and depression, each item is rated on a 4 point scale.
Satisfaction with life scale (SWLS): Diener et al. (1985)	A 5-item scale designed to measure global cognitive judgments of one's life satisfaction. Participants indicate how much they agree or disagree with each of the 5 items using a 7-point scale that ranges from 7 strongly agree to 1 strongly disagree.
Social support questionnaire: Sarason et al. (1983)	A 27-item questionnaire designed to measure perceptions of social support and satisfaction with that social support. Each item is a question that solicits a two-part answer: Part 1 asks participants to list all the people that fit the description of the question, and Part 2 asks participants to indicate how satisfied they are, in general, with these people.
Burns specific health scale (BSHS): Blades et al. (1982)	This questionnaire was designed to assess the post-injury adjustment by means of health-related quality of life in adult burn survivors. It includes both physical and psychosocial domains.

Diabetic Foot Ulcer (DFU)

Diabetes is a widespread and increasingly prevalent condition across the globe with foot ulcers being a common, serious and costly complication experiences by sufferers (Londahl et al. 2011). Diabetic Foot Ulcers (DFUs) are often slow to heal, are associated with increased risk of amputation and death and are costly to treat, with costs to the UK health services estimated to be over £220 million per annum (Majid et al. 2000). Such foot ulcerations have a number of consequences for the individual including reduced mobility and an incapability to perform daily activities. Furthermore, given that the treatment of diabetes-related foot disease demands a multi-disciplinary approach with treatments that are often intensive and prolonged frequent hospitalisations may result (Hogg et al. 2012). These consequences can subsequently negatively impact upon a patient's quality of life. Not only do these, like the other wounds discussed, impact on a patient's physical functioning, but also on their social and psychological status (Londahl et al. 2011). Much research has highlighted these consequences with patients often reporting reduced mobility as a major factor impinging on their QoL (Hogg et al. 2012; Chapman et al. 2014; Ribu and Wahl 2004), followed by having to adapt to the lifestyle changes needed to live with ulcerations on the foot.

A number of studies have reported that individuals with diabetic foot ulcers are faced with a variety of negative emotional and psychological consequences. Research has highlighted how due to the lack of mobility, many patients are faced with feelings of frustration, anger and guilt (Brod 1998; Kinmond et al. 2002; Watson-Miller 2006). These feelings often stem from the restrictions patients perceive. It is important to note that these are often perceptions rather than reality and it is therefore incumbent on the clinician to ensure that appropriate education and support is provided to the patient, along with any practical remedies to improve their mobility.

Not surprisingly, those individuals with DFU have significantly poorer psychosocial states than those with diabetes but without a foot ulcer (Fejfarova et al. 2014). Indeed, Fejfarova et al. (2014) reported that those with a DFU had a lower quality of life in key areas: finances, standard of living, employment status, isolation and financial hardship. Similarly, there were reports of lower levels of social support and self-care. Not surprisingly, levels of suicidal ideation were also relatively high (approximately 5 %).

Other research has also highlighted a high prevalence of depression amongst those with a DFU. For example, phenomenological research conducted by Kinmond et al. (2002) interviewed a number of patients who had an ulceration.

In this study, it was found that almost all of the patients reported negative implications on their social roles and activities. However, in addition to this, patients described how such restrictions led to significant and prolonged periods of clinical depression, to the point where the patient pleaded with clinicians to have an amputation. Such consequences of living with a foot ulcer can be detrimental to both the quality of life and well-being of patients (as we will see later in the book), continuing the vicious circle of reduced wound healing. Hence, it is essential that clinicians are aware of not only the physical and social implications, but also the psychological and emotional toll such illnesses have. In effect, clinicians must adopt multi-faceted treatment regimes in order to assess patients and provide the most effective treatment and delivery of care.

Importantly, psychological morbidity is increased in those with diabetes and DFU by at least two-fold (Anderson et al. 2001; Ali et al. 2006; Carrington et al. 1996). Both depression and anxiety have been reported in those with DFU (Ali et al. 2006) and these can lead to significant issues with self-care. For example, there may be a general neglect in those with depression. Anxiety itself can manifest in range of disorders including generalised anxiety disorders, obsessive-compulsive disorders, PTSD and panic disorders (Lin et al. 2008). Williams et al. (2010) reported that depression in those with type 2 diabetes was associated with twice the rate of a first DFU and, furthermore, a higher rate of amputation (Williams et al. 2011). Additionally, depression in first DFU is associated with a two-fold increase of mortality over 5 years (Ismail et al. 2007). This psychological comorbidity, particularly depression, can lead to additional risks on patients with diabetes and diabetic foot ulcers resulting in poorer self-care and poorer outcomes (Lustman et al. 2000). In contrast, in those with anxiety it has been argued that its link with self-care and clinical outcomes are less clear: dependent on the nature of the anxiety problem, poorer or even enhanced self-care many emerge (DiMatteo et al. 2000).

It is not just psychological distress that may lead to impairment in healing. Vedhara et al. (2010) reported that ineffective coping with the DFU delayed healing with their results suggesting that promoting "effective coping could significantly improve healing rates" (p. 1596). They described confrontational coping as the least effective and related to delayed healing. This coping style is characterised by more controlling, competitive and extroverted. These patients are therefore more likely to challenge the advice of health care professionals and be less willing to follow treatment recommendations. Thus, if these coping techniques could be improved then so could healing- a role for psychological interventions.

Importantly, if the psychological issues can be addressed then there may be an improvement in outcome- both psychologically and medically. Education by itself may not necessarily improve patient self-care although motivational interviewing shows promise in developing patient skills (Gabbay et al. 2011). Given that the single greatest risk factor for DFU is a previous ulceration or amputation (Boulton et al. 2005), with just over a third of patients re-ulcerating within 12 months, interventions are required that can improve self-care, reduce psychological distress and promote protective psychosocial resources (Hunt 2011). In contrast to the limited educational interventions, Vedhara et al. (2012) developed and evaluated a multi-modal psychosocial intervention aimed at modifying potential psychosocial risk factors associated with foot re-ulceration in diabetes (see Fig. 5.2).

Delivered by a specialist diabetic nurse and podiatrist following CBT training, the intervention consisted of weekly 60–90 min sessions for the first 10 weeks, followed by 3 bimonthly maintenance sessions commencing 2 months after the initial phase completion. The intervention was based on the model described in Fig. 5.2 and was designed to achieve the behavioural, emotional, cognitive and social goals outlined with a view to delaying the onset of further DFU development. The results of the study revealed that the participants found the intervention effective and changed their behaviour positively. Whether there was any impact on re-ulceration is yet to be determined. However, the benefits of group interventions for those with potential DFU re-ulceration is evidenced and may support other studies with other wound types (see Chap. 8).

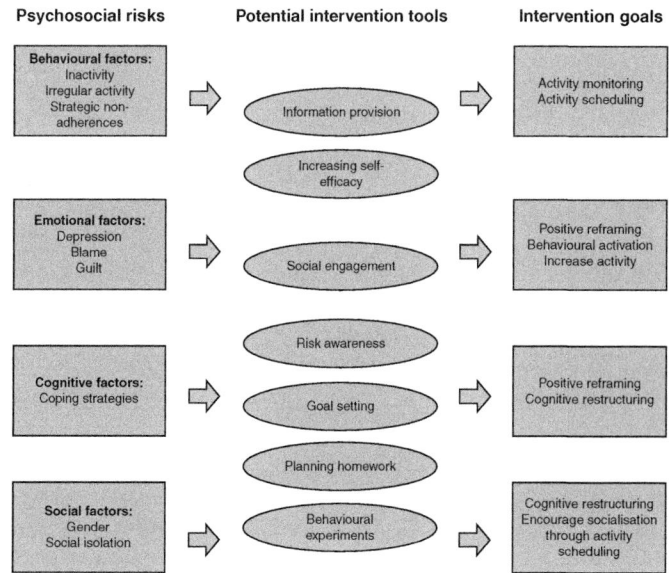

FIGURE 5.2 Conceptual model summarising Vedhara et al. (2012) model of psychosocial factors influencing re-ulceration risk

A final point of note, is that it may not just be the presence of a DFU that leads to psychological distress- this may be apparent in those with a history of DFU but with no current ulcer. In view of the significant behavioural changes that have to be made by the patient to minimise the risk of re-ulceration then there may be an expectation of psychological distress in such individuals. Beattie et al. (2012) interviewed patients who were ulcer free but living with the risk of re-ulceration. Results revealed that most participants experienced a lack of control in preventing further DFUs and this seemed to underpin their psychological and emotional experience. Indeed, there was a high level of depressed mood-surprising given that participants were ulcer free at the time. It is, of course, worrying that such emotional and behavioural responses may serve to increase the risk of developing further ulcers: and that their lack of perceived control appears to be central to these responses. However, these psychosocial risk factors may be ignored or over-looked given that the wound has healed and the perception from health care professionals that no further support is required. There is therefore a need for psychological support for those both with an active ulcer and those with a potential for re-ulceration.

Venous Leg Ulcers

Leg ulceration affects a large number of people within the UK and worldwide, predominantly as a consequence of chronic venous insufficiency (Green and Jester 2009). Annual costs to the NHS, of the reported 70,000–190,000 sufferers are estimated to be some £200 million (Posnett and Franks 2007). Despite both the prevalence and the personal and psychological cost of leg ulcerations on patients, it continues to be misunderstood, often being overlooked and underestimated (Rich and McLachlan 2003). Research surrounding chronic venous leg ulceration demonstrates, unequivocally, the long-term suffering patient's experience that fundamentally impacts upon their quality of life (the importance, of which, will be discussed later in the book; Franks and Moffatt 2001; Maddox 2012). As discussed previously, psychological consequences of living with wounds can include a variety of issues stemming from the pain experiences due to the wound or the isolation that a patient may experience due to living with a wound. Research has highlighted a number of issues associated with living with chronic venous leg ulcers, including pain, leakage of exudate and associated odour, altered body image, reduced mobility, and discomfort associated with wearing bulky bandages. These physical problems can lead to social isolation and psychological dysfunction (Ebbeskog and Ekman 2001a, b; Rich and McLachlan 2003; Hopkins 2004a, b; Ebbeskog and Emami 2005; Jones et al. 2006; Edwards et al. 2009; Green and Jester 2009; Maddoxs 2012; Jones et al. 2008a, b; Moffatt et al. 2009). Hence, it is important for clinicians to understand the predominance of such issues in order to account for such factors within their care procedures.

Green et al. (2013) suggested that VLU had a "pervasive and profound effect" on the daily lives of their participants, with the impact on physical, psychological and social functioning being

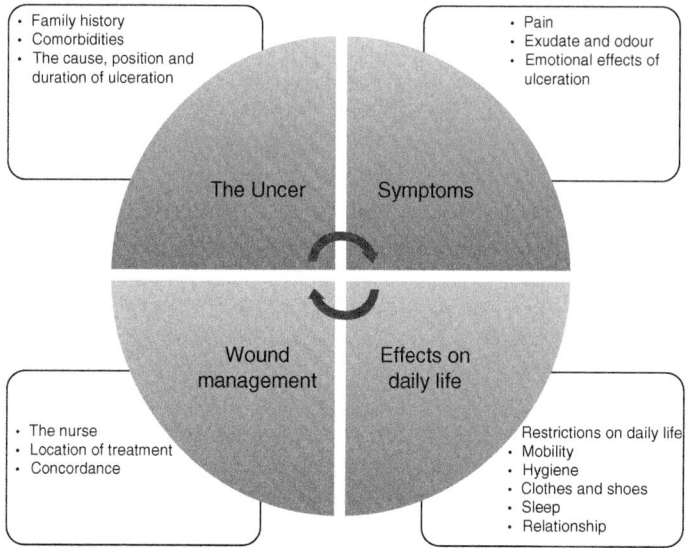

FIGURE 5.3 Four themes underpinning impact of VLU

overwhelming. They suggested that the impact of VLUs could be conceptualised in the model presented in Fig. 5.3.

Qualitative research has highlighted the substantial impact that pain has on the patient's experience. For example, Walshe (1995) conducted semi-structured interviews with patients suffering from venous leg ulcers. Within these interviews, it was reported that pain profoundly affected the life of the patient due to it acting as a constant reminder of their ulceration and, in turn, produced feelings of a loss of control. Similarly, Ebbeskog and Ekman (2001a, b) found that in highlighting pain as a central factor in their daily lives, patients believed it to be a controlling aspect of their lives often making them have feelings of anger and sadness, often resulting in tears. Such emotions are particularly important in assessing patients, particularly when considering the association of such affects with the onset of depression and anxiety, as illustrated above. Another consequence reported as a result of pain is the restrictions often experienced by patients in relation to daily living and physical functioning (Walshe 1995). Reduced mobility was has also been attributed to physical complications of wounds such as leakage of exudate and malodour. For example, research conducted by Rich and McLachlan (2003) highlighted patient's concern surrounding their exudate, often considering it to be unbearable with methods of odour management being inadequate. These complications often leave patients feeling isolated due to self-imposing restrictions that resulted in them being housebound (Walshe 1995). Often patient's concerns surrounding the odour associated with their wound led to increased self-consciousness and subsequent restricted social interactions. Hence, social contact may be significantly reduced. This can have a significant impact upon the psychological health of patients, particularly when considering research highlighting the link between ulcerations, exudate and depression. For example, a direct correlation between problematic exudate, malodour and depression and anxiety has been discovered in relation to venous leg ulcers (Jones et al. 2008a, b). Hence, it is essential for clinicians to assess patient's needs holistically, providing appropriate treatment, advice and support.

Additionally, such social isolation may be sustained by participants' inability to maintain personal hygiene, subsequently impacting on their well-being (Douglas 2001; Ebbeskog and Ekman 2001a, b). Due to such issues, patients have reported excluding themselves from public in order to avoid embarrassment related to the odour emanating from the wound (Rich and McLachlan 2003). Such self-imposed exclusion can often lead to patient's limiting contact to close family and friends (Ebbeskog and Ekman 2001a, b). Findings such as these can be linked to the concept of 'biographical disruption' (Hopkins 2004a, b), whereby distinctions are made between life before and life after ulcerations. Such 'biographical disruption' is distinguished by a negative impact on both the patient's physical and social activity. However, despite the negative affect occurring in relation to living with ulcerations, patients also display hope for future life expectations (Hopkins 2004a, b). Hyde et al. (1999), for example, also reported patients to display an inner strength that encompassed a determination to cope with the ulceration through resilience and hope, particularly related to the healing of their ulcers.

The results of these studies are in line with other studies (e.g. Ebbeskog and Ekman 2001a, b), and in some cases the health care professional (particularly the community nurse) was essential in developing social interaction. The leg club model of leg ulcer management (Lindsay 2001) aims to address the psychosocial aspects of living with a chronic venous leg ulcer and will be explored further in Chap. 8.

Morgan and Moffatt (2008) explored the relationship between patients and the community nurses caring for them. The importance of the nurse-patient relationship was stressed, particularly in developing effective strategies for daily living. However, patients often felt that nurses showed a lack of understanding and a gap was noted between the patient goals for comfort and the nurse goal of healing (more information on the nurse-patient relationship is discussed in Chap. 7). Studies (e.g. Douglas 2001) have highlighted the issues of recurrent problems included nurses experimenting with various dressings and patients receiving conflicting advice about management of their leg ulcer. Furthermore, patients felt that the pain assessment and management issues were not adequately addressed during the consultation. This is important, given that most studies have indicated that pain is the fundamental issue of living with VLU (e.g. Green et al. 2013; see Chap. 2). Pain assessment is essential with all wounds, irrespective of cause and it is interesting to note that the terms and pain descriptors used by patients may differ dependent on the wound (see Table 5.2).

Pressure Ulcers

Pressure ulcers have become an increasing healthcare problem in many countries (Kaltenthaler et al. 2001). Also known as pressure sores, bedsores and decubitus ulcers, these wounds are often found in individuals who are older, neurologically compromised, have mobility problems, seriously ill, or have nutritional deficiencies (Spilsbury et al. 2006a, b). Pressure

TABLE 5.2 Sensory pain descriptors for chronic wounds

Pressure ulcer	Venous ulcer	Arterial ulcer	Mixed ulcer
Tender	Itchy	Tender	Tender
Sharp	Tender	Stinging	Itchy
Throbbing	Throbbing	Sharp	Sore
Aching	Burning	Hurting	Throbbing
Hot burning	Stinging		
Stabbing			
Heavy			
Shooting			

After Gorecki et al. (2011)

Ulcers range in size and severity although the majority are below the waist with particularly vulnerable areas being the sacrum, buttocks and heels. These common wounds are widespread in both hospital and community settings and can have a significant impact on quality of life by compromising many areas of functioning (Gorecki et al. 2010).

There are varying degrees of ulceration that can be classified accordingly (see Table 5.3). As can be seen from the brief descriptions in Table 5.3 the physical consequences of pressure ulcers can be severe and it is not surprising that the financial and psychological costs are significant. Research has highlighted the cost such wounds has on both the UK health and social care system (Bennett et al. 2004). As such, the clinical guidelines published by the National Institute for Health and Clinical Excellence (NICE 2003a, b, 2005) highlight the importance of the prevention and management of pressures ulcers, making treatment, management and care key responsibilities for wound clinicians. As discovered with other wounds, the long-term suffering patient's may experience due to pressure ulcers can have fundamental and significant consequences on their quality of life. Additionally, patients may experience a number of psychological consequences in connection with their ulcerations. However, due to the commonalty that patient's suffering with pressure ulcers are often presented with another debilitating condition, it is somewhat difficult to consider the

Table 5.3 Pressure ulcer and skin classification scale (http://www.npuap.org)

Category/stage	Brief description
Category/stage I	**Non-blanchable erythema**. Intact skin with non-blanchable redness of a localized area usually over a bony prominence. May indicate "at risk" persons.
Category/stage II	**Partial thickness**. Partial thickness loss of dermis presenting as a shallow open ulcer with a red pink wound bed, without slough. This category should not be used to describe skin tears, tape burns, incontinence associated dermatitis, maceration or excoriation
Category/stage III	**Full thickness skin loss**. Full thickness tissue loss. Subcutaneous fat may be visible but bone, tendon or muscle are *not* exposed.
Category/stage IV	**Full thickness tissue loss**. Full thickness tissue loss with exposed bone, tendon or muscle.

impact of such ulcers separate from the impact of other conditions. Nonetheless, research has tried to explore this area.

One phenomenological study considering the lived experiences of eight individuals with either existing or healed pressure ulcers, discovered particularly important negative consequences in association with pressure ulcers (Langemo et al. 2000). Not only did these findings reveal physical, social and financial constraints, but patient's revealed how living with pressure ulcers led to a negative body image, feelings of lack of control (helplessness) and of independence. Similar to previous findings on wounds, Fox (2002) discovered a number of negative consequences stemming from pressure ulcers. These included pain, wound exudation, loss of independence, worries connected with healing, relationship issues, social isolation and reduced body image satisfaction.

One of the key issues for those with the pressure ulcers is pain (Gorecki et al. 2009; Rastinehad 2006; Reddy et al. 2003a, b; Szor and Bourguignon 1999; Gorecki et al. 2010), although according to a literature review (Girouard et al. 2008) it is poorly understood and highlighted the complexity and difficulty in its assessment (see also Chap. 2). PU associated pain can be disabling and interfere with their ability to undertake daily activities and having a detrimental impact on psychological well-being (Gorecki et al. 2009). Interestingly, the descriptive words used to describe pain associated with the different stages of pressure ulcers (see Table 5.3) demonstrated some significant similarities and differences. Hence, sensory words were used by all patients irrespective of PU category. Common words across all Categories II-IV included tender, hurting, burning, sharp, throbbing, hot burning, and aching. Words common for PU Categories II and III included sore; for Categories II and IV: itching and stinging; for Category III and IV: stabbing and heavy (Gorecki et al. 2011).

A model that integrated both the psychosocial variables associated with pain along with the physiological was proposed by Gorecki et al. (2011) which included five main conceptual domains: communicating the pain, feeling the pain, impact of the pain, self-management behaviours, and professional pain management. Importantly, the model suggests that the pain must be managed appropriately both by traditional medical and nursing means but also by effective communication with the patient: "We need to help tissue viability and community nurses link in with other pain management systems to enable them to engage with patients holistically and provide the most effective PU pain management" (p. 456).

Spilsbury et al. (2006a, b) found that pressure ulcer sufferers reported feeling as though they were a burden due to their increasing dependency on others to care for them. This resulted in patient's expressing resentment and frustration at their incapability and need of consistent help. In relation to the impact of pressure ulcers in patients who had suffered traumatic and debilitating injuries (i.e. road accident), such ulcers were considered unimportant. However, other patients became preoccupied over their ulcers, resulting in increased pain and feelings of anxiety whenever anticipating moving positions. This led to further worry associated with the healing of the wounds. As such, patients suffered with feelings of misery and depression. As with the wounds discussed previously the physical and social implications associated with the pressure ulcers often led to a significant psychological impact upon the patients. Thus, it is imperative that clinicians consider such aspects within their care. Further to this, it is important to consider the forms of treatment given to patients, whilst also taking into account the importance they place on their forms of care and management.

Given the significant issues that individuals suffering from pressure ulcers suffer it is not surprising that the levels of Health-Related Quality of Life is compromised (Gorecki et al. 2010, 2012). Indeed several models of HRQL have been developed exploring the relationship between individual components such as symptoms, physical functioning and well-being (e.g. Patrick and Bergner 1990; Fung and Hays 2008). Interestingly, Gorecki et al. (2012) detailed that pressure ulcers directly impact on HRQoL but there were also a range of factors that may intervene to modify this relationship. Of particular importance were the experience of care factors, which appeared to have a direct effect on satisfaction with care and HRQoL.

References

Ali S, Stone MA, Peters JL, Davies MJ, Khunti K. The prevalence of co-morbid depression in adults with type 2 diabetes: a systematic review and meta-analysis. Diabet Med. 2006;23(11): 1165–73.

Anderson RJ, Freedland KE, Clouse RE, Lustman PJ. The prevalence of comorbid depression in adults with diabetes: a meta-analysis. Diabetes Care. 2001;24:1069–78.

Beattie AM, Vedhara K, Metcalfe C, Weinman J, Cullum N, Price P, Dayan C, Cooper A, Campbell R, Chalder T. Development and preliminary evaluation of a psychosocial intervention for modifying psychosocial risk factors associated with foot re-ulceration in diabetes. Behav Res Ther. 2012;50(5):323–32.

Beck AT, Ward CH, Mendelson M, Mock J, Erbaugh J. An inventory for measuring depression. Arch Gen Psychiatry. 1961;4:561–71.

Bennett G, Dealey C, Posnett J. The cost of pressure ulcers in the UK. Age Ageing. 2004;33(3):230–5.

Blades B, Mellis N, Munster AM. A burn specific health scale. J Trauma. 1982;22(10):872–5.

Blalock SJ, Bunker BJ, DeVellis RF. Measuring health status among survivors of burn injury: revisions of the Burn Specific Health Scale. J Trauma Acute Care Surg. 1994;36(4):508–15.

Boulton AJM, Vileikyte L, Ragnarson-Tennvall G, Apelqvist J. The global burden of diabetic foot disease. Lancet. 2005;366:1721–5.

Brod M. Quality of life issues in patients with diabetes and lower extremity ulcers: patients and care givers. Qual Life Res. 1998;7:365–72.

Bryant RA. Predictors of post-traumatic stress disorder following burns injury. Burns. 1996;22(2):89–92.

Cardena E, Koopman C, Classen C, Waelde LC, Spiegel D. Psychometric properties of the Stanford Acute Stress Reaction Questionnaire (SASRQ). J Trauma Stress. 2000;13:719–34.

Carrington AL, Mawdsley SK, Morley M, Kincey J, Boulton AJ. Psychological status of diabetic people with or without lower limb disability. Diabetes Res Clin Pract. 1996;32:19–25.

Carver CS. You want to measure coping but your protocol's too long: consider the brief COPE. Int J Behav Med. 1997;4:92–100.

Carver CS, Scheier MF, Weintraub JK. Assessing coping strategies – a theoretically based approach. J Pers Soc Psychol. 1989;56:267–83.

Chapman Z, Shuttleworth CMJ, Huber JW. High levels of anxiety and depression in diabetic patients with Charcot foot. J Foot Ankle Res. 2014;7(1):22.

Coker AO, Fadeyili OI, Olugbile OG, Zachariah MP, Ademiluyi SA. A psychological morbidity study of patients with major burns seen at a teaching hospital in Lagos, Nigeria. Nig J Plast Surg. 2008;4(2):31–5.

Costa Jr PT, McCrae RR. The NEO personality inventory manual. Odessa: Psychological Assessment Resources; 1985.

Costa Jr PT, McCrae RR. The NEO-PIINEO-FFl manual supplement. Odessa: Psychological Assessment Resources; 1989.

Derogatis L, Melisaratos N. The brief symptom inventory: an introductory report. Psychol Med. 1983;13:595–605.

De Young AC, Kenardy JA, Cobham VE, Kimble R. Prevalence, comorbidity and course of trauma reactions in young burn-injured children. J Child Psychol Psychiatry. 2012;53(1):56–63.

Diener E, Emmons RA, Larsen RJ, Griffin S. The satisfaction with life scale. J Pers Assess. 1985;49:71–5.

DiMatteo MR, Lepper H, Croghan TW. Depression is a risk factor for noncompliance with medical treatment e meta-analysis of the effects of anxiety and depression on patient adherence. Arch Intern Med. 2000;14:101–7.

Diver AJ. The evolution of burn fluid resuscitation. Int J Surg. 2008;6(4):345–50.

Douglas V. Living with a chronic leg ulcer: an insight into patients' experiences and feelings. J Wound Care. 2001;10(9):355–60.

Dyster-Aas J, Willebrand M, Wikehult B, Gerdin B, et al. Major depression and posttraumatic stress disorder symptoms following severe burn injury in relation to lifetime psychiatric morbidity. J Trauma. 2008;64(5):1349–56.

Ebbeskog B, Ekman S-L. Elderly persons' experiences of living with venous leg ulcer: living in a dialectical relationship between freedom and imprisonment. Scand J Caring Sci. 2001a;235–243.

Ebbeskog B, Ekman S. Elderly people's experiences: the meaning of living with venous leg ulcer. Eur Wound Manage Assoc J. 2001b;1(1):21–3.

Ebbeskog B, Emami A. Older patients' experience of dressing changes on venous leg ulcers: more than just a docile patient. J Clin Nurs. 2005;14(10):1223–31.

Edwards H, Courtney M, Finlayson K, Shuter P, Lindsay E. A randomised controlled trial of a community nursing intervention: improved quality of life and healing for clients with chronic leg ulcers. J Clin Nurs. 2009;18(11):1541–9.

Edwards R, Smith M, Klick B, Magyar-Russell G, Haythornthwaite J, Holavanahalli R, Patterson D, Blakeney P, Lezotte D, McKibben J, Fauerbach J. Symptoms of depression and anxiety as unique predictors of pain-related outcomes following burn injury. Ann Behav Med. 2007;34(3):313–22.

Esselman PC, Thombs BD, Magyar-Russell G, Fauerbach JA. Burn rehabilitation: state of the science. Am J Phys Med Rehabil. 2006;85:383–413. doi:10.1097/01.phm.0000202095.51037.a3.

Ewing JA. Detecting alcoholism The CAGE questionnaire. JAMA. 1984;252(14):1905–7.

Fauerbach JA, Lawrence J, Haythornthwaite J, Richter D, McGuire M, Schmidt C, Munster A. Preburn psychiatric history affects posttrauma morbidity. Psychosomatics. 1997;38(4):374–85.

Fauerbach JA, Lezotte D, Hills RA, Cromes GF, Kowalske K, deLateur BJ, Goodwin CW, Blakeney P, Herndon DN, Wiechman SA, Engrav LH, Patterson DR. Burden of burn: a norm-based inquiry into the influence of burn size and distress on recovery of physical and psychosocial function. J Burn Care Rehabil. 2005;26(1):21–32.

Fauerbach JA, McKibben J, Bienvenu OJ, Magyar-Russell G, Smith MT, Holavanahalli R, Patterson DR, Wiechman SA, Blakeney P, Lezotte D. Psychological distress after major burn injury. Psychosom Med. 2007;69(5):473–82.

Fejfarova V, Jirkovska A, Dragomirecka E, et al. Does the diabetic foot have a significant impact on selected psychological or social characteristics of patients with diabetes mellitus. J Diabetes Res. 2014;7.

Foa EB, Riggs DS, Dancu CV, Rothbaum BO. Reliability and validity of a brief instrument for assessing post-traumatic stress disorder. J Trauma Stress. 1993;6:459–73.

Fox C. Living with a pressure ulcer: a descriptive study of patients' experiences. Br J Community Nurs. 2002;7(6 Suppl):10–22.

Franks P, Moffatt C. Health related quality of life in patients with venous ulceration: Use of the Nottingham health profile. Qual Life Res. 2001;10:693–700.

Fung CH, Hays RD. Prospects and challenges in using patient-reported outcomes in clinical practice. Qual Life Res. 2008;17: 1297–302.

Gabbay RA, Kaul S, Ulbretcht J, Scheffer NM, Armstrong DG. Motivational interviewing by podiatric physicians: a method for improving patient self-care of the diabetic foot. J Am Podiatr Med Assoc. 2011;101:78–84.

Gilboa D, Bisk L, Montag I, Tsur H. Personality traits and psychosocial adjustment of patients with burns. J Burn Care Rehabil. 1999a;20(4):340–6.

Gilboa D, Bisk L, Montag I, Tsur H. Personality traits and psychosocial adjustment of patients with burns. J Burn Care Rehabil. 1999b;20(4):340–6.

Girouard K, Harrison MB, VanDenKerkof E. The symptom of pain with pressure ulcers: a review of the literature. Ostomy Wound Manage. 2008;54(5):30–40.

Gorecki C, Brown JM, Nelson EA, Briggs M, Schoonhoven L, Dealey C, et al. Impact of pressure ulcers on quality of life in older patients: a systematic review. J Am Geriatr Soc. 2009;57(7):1175–83.

Gorecki C, Lamping DL, Brown JM, et al. Development of a conceptual framework of health-related quality of life in pressure ulcers: A patient-focused approach. Int J Nurs Stud. 2010;47:1525–34.

Gorecki C, Closs SJ, Nixon J, Briggs M. Patient-reported pressure ulcer pain: a mixed-methods systematic review. J Pain Symptom Manage. 2011;42(3):443–59.

Gorecki C, Nixon J, Madill A, Firth J, Brown JM. What influences the impact of pressure ulcers on health-related quality of life? A qualitative patient-focused exploration of contributory factors. J Tissue Viability. 2012;21:3–12.

Green J, Jester R. Health-related quality of life and chronic venous leg ulceration: part 1. Wound Care. 2009;14(12):12–7.

Green J, Jester R, McKinley R, Pooler A. Patient perspectives of their leg ulcer journey. J Wound Care. 2013;22(2):58–66.

Hammarberg M. Penn inventory for posttraumatic stress disorder: psychometric properties. Psychol Assess. 1992;4(1):67–76.

Herndon D. Total burn care. Philadelphia: Saunders; 2007.

Hodder K, Chur-Hansen A, Parker A. A thematic study of the role of social support in the body image of burn survivors. Health Psychol Res. 2014;2:21–3.

Hogg F, et al. Measures of health-related quality of life in diabetes-related foot disease: a systematic review. Diabetologia. 2012;55(3):552–65.

Hopkins A. Disrupted lives: investigating coping strategies for non-healing leg ulcers. Br J Nurs. 2004a;13(9):556–63.

Hopkins A. The use of qualitative research methodologies to explore leg ulceration. J Tissue Viability. 2004b;14(4):142–7.

Hunt DL. Diabetes: foot ulcers and amputations. Clin Evid (Online). 2011: pii: 0602.

Hyde C, Ward B, Horsfall J, Winder G. Older women's experience of living with chronic leg ulceration. Int J Nurs Pract. 1999;5:189–98.

Ismail K, Winkley K, Stahl D, et al. A cohort study of people with diabetes and their first foot ulcer: the role of depression on mortality. Diabetes Care. 2007;30:1473–9.

Jones J, Barr W, Robinson J, Carlisle C. Depression in patients with chronic venous ulceration. Br J Nurs. 2006;15(11):17–23.

Jones JE, Robinson J, Barr W, Carlisle C. Impact of exudate and odour from chronic venous leg ulceration. Nurs Stand. 2008a;22(45):53–61.

Jones RA, Taylor AG, Bourguignon C. Family interactions among African American Prostate Cancer Survivors. Fam Community Health. 2008b;31(3):213–20.

Kaltenthaler E, Whitfield MD, Walters SJ, Akehurst RL, Paisley S. UK, USA and Canada: how do their pressure ulcer prevalence and incidence data compare? J Wound Care. 2001;10:530–5.

Kildal M, Andersson G, Fugl-Meyer AR, Lannerstam K, Gerdin B. Development of a brief version of the Burn Specific Health Scale (BSHS-B). J Trauma. 2001;51(4):740–6.

Kinmond K, McGee P, Gough S, Ashford R. 'Loss of self': a psychosocial study of the quality of life of adults with diabetic ulceration. 2002. Available at http://www.worldwidewounds.com/2003/may/Kinmond/Loss-Of-Self.html.

Klinge K, Chamberlain DJ, Redden M, King L. Psychological adjustments made by postburn injury patients: an integrative literature review. J Adv Nurs. 2009;65(11):2274–92.

Langemo DK, Melland H, Hanson D, Olson B, Hunter S. The lived experience of having a pressure ulcer: a qualitative analysis. Adv Skin Wound Care. 2000;13(5):225–35.

Lin EH, Korff MV, Alonso J. Mental disorders among persons with diabetes results from the World Mental Health Surveys. J Psychosom Res. 2008;65:571–80.

Lindsay ET. Compliance with science: benefits of developing community leg clubs. Br J Nurs. 2001;10(22 Suppl):S66–74.

Londahl M, Landin-Olsson M, Katzman P. Hyperbaric oxygen therapy improves health-related quality of life in patients with diabetes and chronic foot ulcer. Diabetes Med. 2011;2:186–90.

Lustman PJ, Anderson RJ, Freedland KE, de Groot M, Carney RM, et al. Depression and poor glycemic control: a meta-analytic review of the literature. Diabetes Care. 2000;23:934–42.

Maddox D. Effects of venous leg ulceration on patients' quality of life. Nurs Stand. 2012;26(38):42–9.

Majid M, Cullum N, Fletcher A, O'Meara S, Sheldon T. Systematic reviews of wound care management: diabetic foot ulcers. Health Technol Assess. 2000;4:1–237.

Mendelson BK, Mendelson MJ, White DR. Body-esteem scale for adolescents and adults. J Pers Assess. 2001;76(1):90–106.

Moffatt C, Kommala D, Dourdin N, Choe Y. Venous leg ulcers: patient concordance with compression therapy and its impact on healing and prevention of recurrence. Int Wound J. 2009;6:386–93.

Morgan PA, Moffatt CJ. Non healing leg ulcers and the nurse–patient relationship. Part 2: the nurse's perspective. Int Wound J. 2008;5(2):332–9.

Munster AM, Moran KT, Thupari J, Allo M, Winchurch RA. Prophylactic intravenous immunoglobulin replacement in high risk burn patients. J Burn Care Rehabil. 1987;8:376–80.

NICE. Pressure ulcer prevention. London: National Institute for Health and Clinical Excellence; 2003a. Available at: http://www.nice.org.uk/page.aspx?o¼CG007NICEguideline.

NICE. Pressure ulcer risk assessment and prevention, including the use of pressure-relieving devices (beds, mattresses and overlays) for the prevention of pressure ulcers in primary and secondary care. National Institute for Health and Clinical Excellence. London. 2003b. Available at: www.nice.org.uk/page.aspx?o=20052.

NICE. Pressure ulcers: the management of pressure ulcers in primary and secondary care. National Institute for Health and Clinical Excellence. London. 2005. http://www.nice.org.uk/nicemedia/pdf/CG029fullguideline.pdf.

Noronha DO, Faust MS. Identifying the variables impacting post-burn psychological adjustment: a meta-analysis. J Pediatr Psychol. 2006;32(3):380–91.

Norris SL, Gober JR, Haywood LJ, Halls J, Boswell W, Colletti P, Terk M. Altered muscle metabolism shown by magnetic resonance spectroscopy in sickle cell disease with leg ulcers. Magn Reson Imaging. 1993;11:119–23.

Park SH, Cho MS, Kim YS, Hong J, Nam E, Park J, et al. Self-reported health-related quality of life predicts survival for patients with advanced gastric cancer treated with first-line chemotherapy. Qual Life Res. 2008;17(2):207–14.

Partridge J, Robinson E. Psychological and social aspects of burns. Burns. 1995;21(6):453–7.

Patrick DL, Bergner M. Measurement of health status in the 1990's. Annu Rev Public Health. 1990;11:165–83.

Posnett J, Franks PJ. The costs of skin breakdown and ulceration in the UK. In: Pownall M, editor. Skin breakdown: the silent epidemic. Hull: Smith & Nephew; 2007. p. 6–12.

Rastinehad D. Pressure ulcer pain. J Wound Ostomy Continence Nurs. 2006;33(3):252–6.

Reddy M, Kohr R, Queen D, Keast D, Sibbald RG. Practical treatment of wound pain and trauma: a patient-centered approach. An overview. Ostomy Wound Manage. 2003a;49(4 Suppl):2–15.

Reddy M, Keast D, Fowler E, Sibbald RG. Pain in pressure ulcers. Ostomy Wound Manage. 2003b;49(4A Suppl):30–5.

Ribu L, Wahl A. How patients with diabetes who have foot and leg ulcers perceive the nursing care they receive. J Wound Care. 2004;2:65–8.

Rich A, McLachlan L. How living with a leg ulcer affects people's daily life: a nurse-led study. J Wound Care. 2003;12(2):51–4.

Sarason IG, Levine HM, Basham RB, Sarason BR. Assessing social support: the social support questionnaire. J Pers Soc Psychol. 1983;44:127–39.

Smith JS, Smith KR, Rainey SL. The psychology of burn care. J Trauma Nurs. 2006;13(3):105–6.

Spilsbury K, Nelson A, Cullum N, Iglesias C, Nixon J, Mason S. Pressure ulcers and their treatment and effects on quality of life: hospital inpatient perspectives. J Adv Nurs. 2007a;57(5):494–504.

Spilsbury K, Nelson A, Cullum N, Iglesias C, Nixon J, Mason S. Pressure ulcers and their treatment and effects on quality of life: hospital inpatient perspectives. J Adv Nurs. 2007b;57(5):494–504.

Szor JK, Bourguignon C. Description of pressure ulcer pain at rest and at dressing change. J Wound Ostomy Continence Nurs. 1999;26(3):115–20.

Taal LA, Faber AW. Burn injuries, pain and distress: exploring the role of stress symptomatology. Burns. 1997;23(4):288–90.

Van Loey NE, VanSon MJ. Psychopathology and psychological problems in patients with burn scars: epidemiology and management. Am J Clin Dermatol. 2003;4(4):245–72.

Van Loey NE, Van Beeck EF, Faber BW, Van De Schoot R, et al. Health-related quality of life after burns: a prospective multicenter cohort study with 18 months follow-up. J Trauma Acute Care Surg. 2012;72(2):513–20.

Vedhara K, Beattie A, Metcalfe C, Roche S, Weinman J, Cullum N, Price P, Dayan C, Cooper AR, Campbell R, Chalder T. Development and preliminary evaluation of a psychosocial intervention for modifying psychosocial risk factors associated with foot re-ulceration in diabetes. Behav Res Ther. 2012;50:323–32.

Vedhara K, Miles JN, Wetherell MA, Dawe K, et al. Coping style and depression influence the healing of diabetic foot ulcers: observational and mechanistic evidence. Diabetologia. 2010;53(8):1590–8.

Walshe C. Living with a venous leg ulcer: a descriptive study of patients' experiences. J Adv Nurs. 1995;22(6):1092–100.

Watson-Miller S. Living with a diabetic foot ulcer: a phenomenological study. J Clin Nurs. 2006;15:1336–7.

Weiss DS, Marmar CR. The impact of event scale-revised. In: Wilson JP, Keane TM, editors. Assessing psychological trauma and PTSD: a practitioner's handbook. New York: Guilford Press; 1997. p. 399–411.

White CE, Renz EM. Advances in surgical care: management of severe burn injury. Crit Care Med. 2008;36(7):S318–24.

Willebrand M, Kildal M, Ekselius L, Gerdin B, Andersson G. Development of the coping with burns questionnaire. Pers Individ Differ. 2001;30:1059–72.

Williams LH, Rutter CM, Katon WJ, et al. Depression and incident diabetic foot ulcers: a prospective cohort study. Am J Med. 2010;123(8):748–54.

Williams LH, Miller DR, Fincke G, Lafrance JP, Etzioni R, Maynard C, Raugi GJ, Reiber GE. Depression and incident lower limb amputations in veterans with diabetes. J Diabetes Complications. 2011;25:175–82.

Young A. Rehabilitation of burn injuries. Phys Med Rehabil Clin N Am. 2002;13(1):85–108.

Zigmond AS, Snaith RP. The hospital anxiety & depression scale. Acta Psychiatr Scand. 1983;67:361–70.

Chapter 6
Treatment

> Box 6.1: Key Points
> - Treatment for wound care brings with it a range of potential psychological consequences such as pain, embarrassment, stress and body image readjustments;
> - Pain and stress at dressing change can result in physiological changes that may hinder wound healing;
> - It is therefore imperative that the psychological consequences of treatment are fully addressed as doing so may improve wound healing;
> - Different forms of wound management can bring with it different challenges- different dressing types, for example, may be more painful and stressful than others;
> - Increasing concordance to treatment is particularly difficult for a number of reasons, not least the pain, stress and body image adjustment that may result from certain treatments;
> - Different stages of treatment can have different consequences and clinicians should ensure that appropriate assessments are taken throughout the whole process.

Summary

As noted in other chapters, chronic wounds may cause financial, emotional and psychological strain for the patient. However, it is not just the wound that can cause these problems- it may also be the treatment for their wound. This chapter explores some of the psychological issues related to the treatment for chronic wounds, detailing three particular areas of treatment. Firstly, the stresses and strains of dressing change are explored. This highlights how the pain and stress may be associated with the dressing regime and, how, changing to an appropriate dressing choice may reduce both pain and stress. In such a way it may be possible to improve healing by reducing the stress associated with inappropriate dressing technique. Secondly, compression therapy will be explored and how concordance with this may be low and thereby reducing the effectiveness of the treatment. Techniques to improve concordance with treatment will also be explored. Finally, the pain and stress of Negative Pressure Wound Therapy (NPWT) will be outlined and how this may change across the course of treatment- emphasising the need to assess psychological variables throughout the course of any health related intervention.

Introduction

Although many wounds have the potential to become chronic, certain medical conditions are commonly associated with non-healing wounds. These conditions include DFU, chronic venous ulcers, arterial ulcers and pressure ulcers. These pose a significant treatment challenge for the healthcare professional and can result in significant issues for the patient given not only the chronic nature of the wound but also the frequent, and often painful, treatment. The principles of the management of chronic wounds include effective debridement, stimulating the intrinsic process of wound healing and using appropriate dressing techniques until the wound bed is ready for wound closure. Each of these elements has the potential to cause significant issues for the patient.

It is well recognised that the chronic wound care regime can be stressful, painful and socially isolating. The dressing change may have to occur frequently and can result in significant pain and anxiety for the individual patient. In addition there are numerous forms of dressing, elements involved in any dressing change along with a myriad of forms of specialist treatment. Each of these elements may result in concerns, social and psychological issues and potential distress. However, it is obviously impossible to do justice to all of these and as such this chapter will explore just three elements of wound care regimes: the stress and pain involved in dressing change, the use of compression bandages and the use of Negative Pressure Wound Therapy (NPWT).

Dressing Change

Wound pain and stress continue to be an important clinical focus in wound care. In light of this, many consensus documents and statements have been published to provide healthcare professionals with best practice guidance on the management of wound pain (WUWHS 2007). Specifically, the pain caused by the removal of dressings has been identified as a major contributor of wound pain (White 2008), from a patient and healthcare professional perspective (Price et al. 2008b; Kammerlander and Eberlein 2002). In particular, a survey by Hollinworth and Collier (2000) indicated that healthcare professionals were aware of the importance of preventing pain during wound care, however they were unaware of the types of dressings that can be used to minimise this. It has been suggested that patients with wounds should have an individual pain management plan, including regular review and reassessment (Solowiej et al. 2010a, b). It is therefore important that particular attention is paid to dressing selection for patients on an individual basis, as it is known that poor dressing choice can lead to increased wound pain.

Wound dressings have often been classified in simplistic terms, with reference to the interaction that takes place

TABLE 6.1 Three main categories of wound dressing

Dressing adherence	Explanation
Adherent	E.g. dressing pads/cotton gauze – able to adhere to any type of drying wound
Low-adherent	E.g. absorbent dressings – designed to reduce adherence to the wound surface
Non-adherent	E.g. hydrocolloids/hydrogels/alginates – dressings that maintain a moist gel layer over the wound to prevent adherence

Adapted from Thomas (2003)

between the wound and the dressing itself – adherence (Thomas 2003) (see Table 6.1).

Traditional dressings such as cotton gauze and bandages were often replaced with more modern technology once clinical research demonstrated that keeping wounds moist was beneficial for wound healing (Rippon et al. 2008). However, even some modern dressings cause skin damage from repeated application and removal, which causes additional skin damage and increased wound pain. More recently a category of wound dressings have been introduced that are designed to minimise the skin trauma and pain caused by removal. Atraumatic dressings present a category of products that do not cause trauma to the wound or surrounding skin on removal and reapplication, thus reducing pain (Thomas 2003). Specifically, atraumatic dressings utilise technologies that have been developed to avoid adhesion, for example soft silicone adhesive technology (Rippon et al. 2008). The term atraumatic can refer to dressings that are adhesive and non-adhesive, coated in soft silicone to interact with dry skin, but not the fragile wound surface. Therefore, it is suggested that careful selection of atraumatic dressings would benefit the wound healing process, as they contribute significantly to a reduction in pain. In support of this, White (2008) demonstrated that the introduction of atraumatic dressings with soft silicone adhesive in replacement of other dressings (including, adhesive foams and hydrocolloids) significantly reduced

TABLE 6.2 Mean psychological and physiological pain and stress scores for patients receiving atraumatic and conventional dressings

Pain/stress measures	Atraumatic Mean (SD)	Conventional Mean (SD)
STAI (State)	37.09 (15.45)	33.55 (11.21)
Numerical pain	1.25 (1.04)	3.76 (3.11)
Numerical stress	1.75 (0.87)	3.74 (2.62)
HR	69.30 (7.13)	75.75 (14.24)
RR	16.70 (7.72)	16.11 (1.97)
Systolic BP	125.36 (11.66)	138.24 (17.05)
Diastolic BP	64.80 (11.79)	69.59 (12.77)
GSR	19.76 (5.42)	33.15 (16.32)
Salivary cortisol	0.14 (0.03)	0.17 (0.10)

further trauma to the skin and wound-associated pain in a large multinational survey of patients with chronic wounds.

In a study by Upton and Solowiej (2012) the impact of dressing type on wound pain and stress was explored. It was hypothesised that patients with atraumatic dressings as part of their treatment regime would experience less pain at dressing change, in comparison with patients who are treated with conventional dressings. It was found that patients being treated with conventional dressings experienced significantly higher numerical pain ratings, numerical stress ratings, along with the physiological measures of stress- systolic BP, and GSR (Galvanic Skin Response)- at dressing change in comparison with the atraumatic dressings group (see Table 6.2).

In addition to the increased physiological indicators of stress amongst patients receiving conventional dressings, the self-reported severity of acute pain and stress also demonstrated higher pain and stress at dressing change for the conventional dressing group (see Fig. 6.1).

Overall, the findings of this research demonstrated that patients receiving atraumatic dressings as part of their

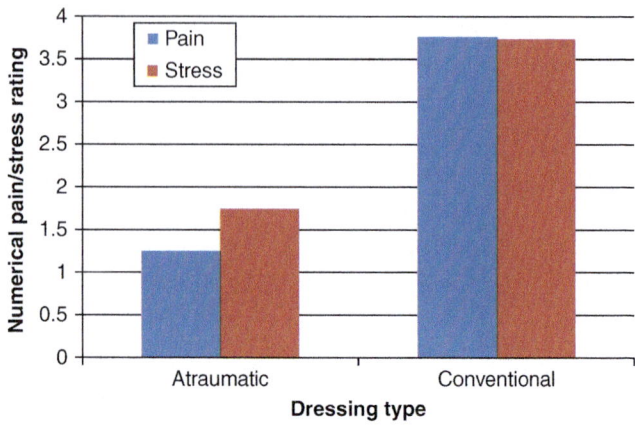

Figure 6.1 Self-reported numerical stress and pain ratings of patients receiving atraumatic and conventional dressings as part of wound treatment

wound treatment experienced significantly lower episodes of acute pain and stress at dressing change in comparison with patients being treated with conventional dressings. In particular, atraumatic dressings appear to improve and minimise the experience of acute stress and pain at dressing change.

Overall, the results of the Upton and Solowiej (2012) study support the notion that appropriate selection of dressings can contribute to a reduction in acute pain and stress, which could lead to an overall improvement in wound treatment experience. A more recent study, reported by Parvaneh et al. (2014) monitored the stress in a group of patients (n=20) continuously whilst they waited for their treatment, underwent a dressing change and then in the post-dressing period. Their results indicated higher stress during the dressing change compared to before the treatment. Unfortunately in this pilot study no comparison between dressing types or wound care regimes was explored but their innovative technique of recording stress through a wearable sensor in real time does open this possibility in the future.

These studies have demonstrated the impact of the dressing type on various psychological measures. Although Upton and Solowiej (2012) explored atraumatic dressings in comparison

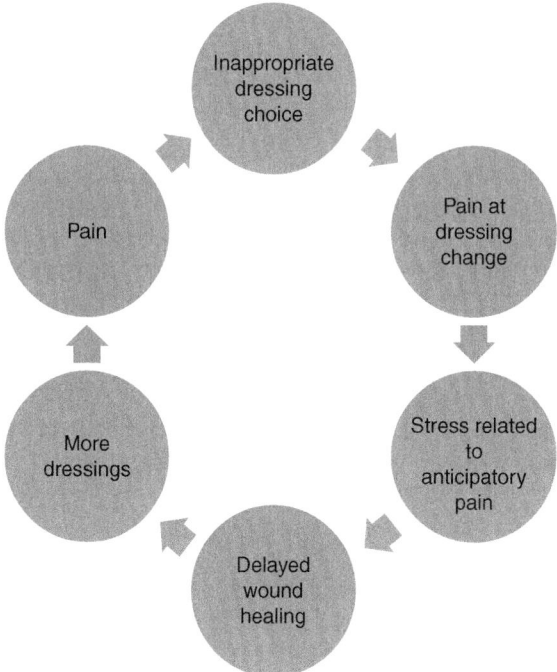

Figure 6.2 Cycle of pain, stress, wound healing, and wound dressing

to other dressings, the nature of the dressing was less relevant than the key message: dressing type can influence stress and pain experienced. Hence, the clinician has to consider the use of *appropriate* dressings for the individual patient. As has been highlighted by many, the choice of dressing should be made on the basis of a clear assessment of the patient and their wound- if the dressing is right for the patient and their wound and can minimise pain then the stress will be ameliorated and healing promoted (see the Fig. 6.2).

Compression Bandaging

For those with leg ulceration of venous aetiology, compression therapy is the gold standard treatment, with compression bandages accelerating ulcer healing when compared with no compression, and multicomponent bandages appearing to be more effective than single layered bandages (O'Meara et al. 2009). However, in 60–70 % of cases, ulcers recur with those that do heal requiring a lifelong plan to prevent recurrence, usually consisting of the on-going use of compression bandages, which imposes a life-long chronic treatment on the individual (Abbade et al. 2005). Moffatt et al. (2009) identified that recurrence rates of wounds were 2–20 times greater when patients did not correctly comply with their prescribed compression bandages suggesting that compliance to treatment is vital for the complete healing of wounds.

Although compression bandages are considered to be the gold standard treatment for venous leg ulcers concordance of them by patients can be poor, which has been noted to be between 48 and 83 % (Moffatt 2004b; Jull et al. 2004a; Van Hecke et al. 2007). Although compression bandages may be considered the cornerstone of venous leg ulcer treatment, this is only if they are fitted correctly and used appropriately. Unfortunately, this is not always the case (Feben 2003; Filed 2004; Todd 2011). This is important as correct application can lead to faster healing times, reduced nursing time and improved patient concordance with treatment (Todd 2011). Indeed, the healing of leg ulcers is largely dependent on the consistency and accuracy of the bandaging technique (Todd 2011). It has been suggested that the right bandaging technique is achieved with experience (Hopkins 2008), however, as Satpathy et al. (2006) identified in their study the correct pressure is often not always achieved even by experienced practitioners. Furthermore, studies have reported that nurses who claim to have experience in applying compression bandages often bandaged in a way that did not produce sustained graduated compression (Feben 2003). Consequently, although there may be a link between experience and accurate technique this is neither linear nor straight-forward. The inaccurate bandaging could lead to delayed healing times, problems relating to ill-fitted bandages and reduced patient concordance with treatment. Furthermore, if the compression is incorrect then there could be poor clinical outcomes for the patient including tissue damage, pain, oedema and necrosis (Todd 2011), which could (obviously) significantly impact patients' overall wellbeing (Milne 2013).

It has also been identified that national guidelines (e.g. RCN 2006; SIGN 1998; CREST 1998) for compression bandaging are not always followed (Sadler et al. 2006; Templeton and Telford 2010). Randell et al. (2009) identified that nurses' decision on which compression dressing to apply usually relied upon past clinical experience with some nurses more than willing to give a particular dressing 'a go'. Additionally, nurses who were interviewed felt as if guidelines for compression bandaging were of limited use to them and their patients and they worked outside of these guidelines for these reasons. It was also noted by Randell et al. (2009) that these guidelines were often prepared by GP's without consultation with the expert nurses who took primary responsibility for caring for those with wounds. This subsequently led to many guidelines never being properly consulted by nurses, and 'bending them' to suit the health care professionals needs.

Research has also suggested reasons for reluctance on the part of nurses to use compression bandages: fear of compression damage; the patient having mobility or footwear issues; problems with patient concordance; and uncertainty over treating mixed aetiology ulcers (Field 2004; Annells et al. 2008; Randell et al. 2009; Todd 2013; Ashby et al. 2014). Furthermore, it is essential that nurses who apply these types of bandages understand the theory behind it and the differences in sub-bandage pressure, failure to do so may lead to longer healing times, pressure damage and even amputation (Todd 2011).

In sum, nurses' understanding of compression bandages, including using the correct compression recommended, the type of compression bandage used, the bandaging technique used, and, indeed, even if nurses decide to use compression bandages, can all impact on their correct use, patient concordance and the patient experience (Feben 2003; Puffett et al. 2006; Annells et al. 2008; Randell et al. 2009; Todd 2013; Ashby et al. 2014).

Compression bandages need to feel firm, especially around the ankle and patients need to be able to move the ankle and foot freely, as a loss of range of motion at the ankle increases an individual's risk of developing ulceration and reduces healing (Barwell et al. 2001). Indeed, it has been recommended that people wear the highest level of compression that is comfortable (Nelson 2012). However in some cases it has been reported that this causes pain for the patient as they are unable to move their toes (Stephen-Haynes 2006). Furthermore, not all patients can tolerate high compression bandages due to the pain and discomfort, and according to some studies, compression bandages can cause pain for patients that can result in poor concordance (Briggs and Flemming 2007; Todd 2011; Weller et al. 2013). For instance, Briggs et al. (2007) found that one participant they interviewed indicated that compression bandages began to cause excessive discomfort and pain that was intolerable and they would contact their clinic immediately to be seen at the earliest time available to review the situation. Furthermore, failure of satisfactory pain relief for the patient caused non-concordance of compression bandages, which resulted in poor patient outcomes. Indeed, Miller et al. (2011) identified that increased pain was a significant predictor of non-concordance with compression bandages.

Additionally, it has been noted that adherence to treatment depends on patient willingness to adapt to treatment regimes. Annells et al. (2008) explored the willingness of patients to comply with compression bandages reporting that one of the reasons for low concordance was that pain caused by either the tightness, or the resultant swelling, from bandages. As well as this, bandages that were uncomfortable for the patient and caused pain can be a constant reminder of the wound and therefore affect the patient's self-image, identity and day-to-day life. Furthermore, Dereure et al. (2005) identified that over 65 % of patients considered applying compression very difficult and 23 % found wearing compression bandages painful. Although multicomponent compression bandages are reported to achieve the best healing rate without pain, research has indicated that this type of bandaging causes pain, and achieving the correct compression is nurse dependent (Anand et al. 2003).

As highlighted, compression bandages are required for as long as there is venous leg ulceration, which may be a lifetime (O'Meara et al. 2009; Moffatt 2004b). Bandages are typically applied from the base of the toes to just below the knee and this may have a significant impact on both an individual's body appearance and their body image. Indeed, a number of studies have suggested that compression bandages may negatively affect body image, appearance and social activity, which may significantly reduce patient concordance with treatment. For example, Annells et al. (2008) suggested that patients decided to stay at home when not being able to wear normal shoes due to bulky bandages or because of the unsightly visibility of the bandages. Similarly, Finlayson et al. (2009) identified that in their sample of 122 patients with venous leg ulcers more than half used padding or covered their legs or avoided going outside or in any situation which may cause any trauma to the legs, which again could lead to social isolation. Furthermore, Dereure et al. (2005) evaluated concordance rates with compression therapy in patients with venous leg ulcers using a questionnaire completed by 1,397 patients. It was identified that 40 % were unable to wear their regular shoes and 45 % regarded compression bandages as unaesthetic which then led to lower concordance to treatment.

Similarly, Mudge et al. (2006) identified that specialist footwear formed a central focus of the patient's body image. Having to wear specialist footwear caused patients embarrassment and consequently affected them going out or socialising This also affected a patient's decision on what to wear, with many feeling that wearing trainers was unacceptable with a skirt, and therefore wore trousers. As well as this the authors found that patients would modify their footwear to accommodate the bandages. Furthermore, King et al. (2007) reported on the views of 102 patients, of which 26 % of patients wore socks, slippers or no foot wear at all due to compression bandages. Thirty- two per cent needed to wear open toe shoes, sandals or slip-ons to be able to wear footwear. Furthermore, some patients wore washable footwear, with others having to wear footwear that was stained. All of these could contribute to reduced patient concordance, as well as restricting individuals to only going out when it was dry, limiting the amount of daily walks they could take, which ultimately may hinder the healing process (Kroger and Assenheimer 2013).

The literature surrounding itching and compression bandages is limited but informative. Annells et al. (2008) identified that some patients removed compression bandages due to itching and dry skin underneath the bandages. However, although removing bandages could offer some relief it could also affect the healing process. Additionally, Edwards (2003) found that compression bandages caused patients to have irritation of the skin, which then lead to scratching behaviours, where some patients would insert objects in between the bandages to scratch the skin. This can again affect the wound by giving the patient additional skin trauma and cause more pain and exudate for the patient, and consequently resulting in low concordance to treatment from patients (Upton et al. 2012b, c).

A number of issues relating to patient experience using compression bandages can be identified. In particular, concordance to treatment advice may be limited for a number of reasons. The pain of the treatment, the inappropriate fitting, mobility problems, and the willingness to adapt to the treatment are all factors that have been reported as being influential in concordance to treatment. This is important whatever the treatment- not just compression therapy. An effective regime relies on appropriate concordance to treatment by the patient, which in itself relies on communication, commitment and expertise by the practitioner. Some of the issues that may face the health care expert have been outlined here, and these have to be acknowledged and addressed by the health care professional in order to improve both concordance and outcomes.

Negative Pressure Wound Therapy

Negative Pressure Wound Therapy (NPWT) also known as VAC (Vacuum Assisted Closure) or Topical Negative Pressure (TNP) is a therapeutic technique, which facilitates the healing of acute and chronic wounds whilst preventing the occurrence of infection (Ubbink et al. 2008). This treatment was first established in the 1980s and developed further in the 1990s to deal with large and complex wounds which posed difficulties when attempting to achieve definitive wound closure (Panicker 2009).

Research has highlighted some benefits associated with NPWT, including; its ease of use for both carers and patients (Stansby et al. 2010), minimal reports of pain (Stansby et al. 2010; Panicker 2009) and significant reduction in wound size. Additionally, Augustin et al. (2006) found that patients using NPWT reported high satisfaction with the treatment. Furthermore, significant improvements were found across multiple areas, including physical symptoms, psychological and social wellbeing, and daily life.

A common complaint of NPWT is pain during dressing change. For example, one study reported that 67 % of patients experienced pain during dressing change when undergoing NPWT for gynaecologic malignancies, despite experiencing no other complications other than bleeding in one patient out of a total of 27 (Schimp et al. 2003). Stansby et al. (2010) who considered pain levels associated with NPWT and its ease of use from the perspective of both patients and carers. Patients reported low levels of pain, with 22 % of patients experiencing pain during treatment activation, 31 % at dressing changes and 17 % at treatment deactivation. The authors concluded that NPWT minimises pain. Furthermore, both patients and carers deemed the NPWT system to be easy to use. However, this study was a non-controlled, clinical investigation; it thus lacked the rigour associated with randomised controlled trials (RCTs).

Despite these findings, high levels of pain were reported in another study (Apostoli and Caula 2008) investigated the impact of NPWT on patients' pain and functional activities. Other studies have also considered ways in which pain can be minimised with NPWT. For example, Wolvos (2004) conducted a retrospective analysis of five cases of patients receiving NPWT and reported that instillation of a topical anaesthetic into the wound reduced pain for people having NPWT.

Additionally, studies have considered the use of low-pressure NPWT and the effects on pain levels. In a case study of two patients with Fournier's Gangrene, average pain scores were reported to be low to moderate during treatment and dressing changes. It was also reported that this type of NPWT was easy to use and promoted patient comfort (Verbelen et al. 2011). Another study exploring low-pressure NPWT in three wound patients found that average pain levels were moderate (4–5 out of 10) and that pain levels tended to reduce during the course of treatment (Nease 2009)

The majority of the studies reported so far did not take measures to explore patients' experiences throughout the treatment intervention. Fixed scoring measures, such as inferring pain through pain-killer dosage, were used in order to report wound pain, odour and ease of dressing changes. Therefore, whilst the findings provide some insight into the pain associated with NWPT, they say little about patients' experience during treatment.

Research focusing on the quality of life (QoL) of patients receiving NPWT has reported mixed findings, although several studies have reported patient benefits of NPWT, such as reduced frequency of dressing changes and less time spent in hospital (Assenza et al. 2011). Bryan and Dukes (2009) reported the case of a 55-year-old woman receiving NPWT who was able to spend time at home rather than in hospital due to the treatment, although the noise of the device impacted upon her ability to sleep, and regular visits to the hospital resulted in her requiring support from family members. However, the patient in this study suffered a bereavement during the process, so this is likely to have affected her life considerably.

Despite such findings, the above studies have not directly explored quality of life in patients receiving NPWT. One study that focused on the impact of NPWT on QoL involved the use of the Cardiff Wound Impact Schedule (CWIS) to measure QoL in 26 patients receiving NPWT (Mendonca et al. 2007). The authors measured QoL before therapy and again 4 weeks after treatment or at wound closure. It was reported that there was no significant change in the QoL of patients whose wounds healed, but that scores on the physical-functioning domain of the CWIS decreased in ambulatory patients, and global QoL worsened for people requiring surgical intervention. The authors concluded that NPWT can cause QoL to worsen in some cases. However, no control group was used and NPWT did not appear to reduce QoL overall.

Other researchers have also used the CWIS to measure QoL in patients receiving NPWT (Ousey et al. 2012). In this study, the authors compared QoL scores of NPWT patients (n=10) with those of patients receiving traditional wound therapies (n=11). No significant differences were found in QoL scores over a 12-week period, showing that QoL was neither better nor worse for NPWT patients overall. However, a surprising finding was that patients who received NPWT showed an improvement on the social life domain of the CWIS in the first 2-weeks. This was not found for patients receiving standard treatment. The authors speculated that this improvement could possibly be due to NPWT patients developing confidence to go out and socialise, or it may have been related to exudates management. However, the authors also acknowledged that there were younger patients in the NPWT group, so these patients may have been keener to socialise.

Wallin et al. (2011) evaluated outcomes of NPWT by analysing clinical data for 87 patients who received NPWT. The authors reported that NPWT was successful in treating wounds for 71 % of patients. However, concerns about QoL resulted in cessation of treatment for four patients. Additionally, equipment difficulties were noted for two patients. This study suggests that NPWT may negatively impact upon the QoL of some patients. However, this was only found for a minority of the patients in the study, and the authors relied on analysing clinical data rather than exploring patients' experiences.

In contrast, another study reported great improvements in the QoL of NPWT patients (Karatepe et al. 2011). The

QoL of patients receiving NPWT was compared with that of patients receiving standard treatment, using the SF-36 questionnaire, which was administered on the day before treatment commencement and then again in the month following wound closure. It was found that healing time was significantly lower in those receiving NPWT and that scores improved considerably on all eight domains of the SF-36, and on the Physical and Mental Component Summaries.

Since anxiety can impact upon patient wellbeing and also on their treatment outcomes, the level of anxiety experienced during treatment needs to be considered. This was investigated in 20 patients undergoing NPWT for traumatic wounds of the lower extremity, compared to 20 patients with similar wounds who were receiving traditional treatment (Keskin et al. 2008). Anxiety measures were taken on the day before NPWT was applied and then on the 10th day of treatment using the Hamilton Rating Scale for Anxiety and the State Anxiety Inventory Test. A significant increase in anxiety was reported for both groups during the 10 day period. However, the mean differences in anxiety scores for the NWPT group over the 10 days were significantly higher than for those receiving standard treatment. This suggests that NPWT can considerably increase patient anxiety levels. However, the authors only looked at a 10-day period, so the findings do not tell us about anxiety levels throughout the NPWT process and after treatment.

In a series of studies, Upton and Andrews (2013a, b, c) reported on the pain and stress associated with NPWT from both a clinician and patient perspective and across the different time points of treatment. Findings from their sample of 50 patients and over 200 clinicians worldwide indicated that the majority rated the experience of NPWT, and the impact of the treatment on their wound, positively. However, it was also clear that NPWT involved a number of challenges for patients. For example, it was found that NPWT affected the mobility, daily activities and sleep of over half the sample. In addition to the various practical difficulties with NPWT, patients also reported experiencing pain during treatment. Whilst the majority of patients did not experience wound pain generally (55 %), a large number of respondents reported experiencing pain during dressing change. Dressing removal

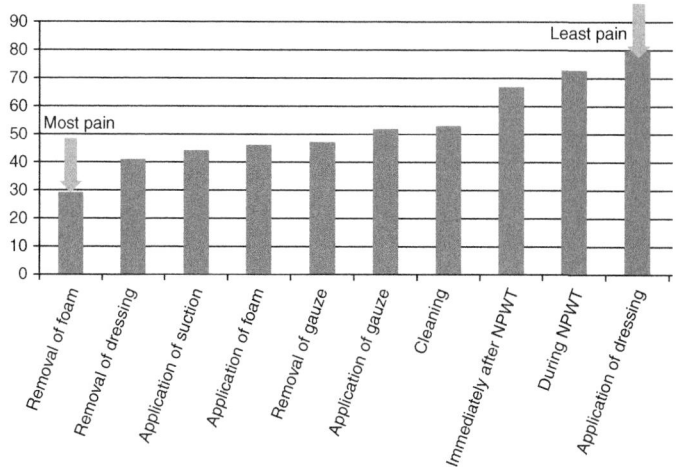

FIGURE 6.3 Clinicians reports of minimal/no pain

was considered to be the most painful stage, with 53 % experiencing some level of pain during this stage, followed by dressing application (49 %). Clinician reports are indicated in Fig. 6.3 and suggest that they considered removal of foam to be the most painful, with the application of the dressing the least painful. Given the changes over time, these findings indicate that accurate pain assessment is needed throughout the stages of NPWT so as to ensure appropriate support is given.

The experiences of patients in these studies suggested that pain is greatest at the beginning of treatment, during the initial dressing changes. In a similar way, respondents also stated that stress or anxiety in relation to NPWT tended to be greatest at the start and to reduce over time (however, somewhat different to the Parvaneh et al. (2014) study that reported greater stress at dressing change compared to prior to dressing change). Over a third of patients had experienced some anxiety during NPWT, with others suggesting that stress had occurred early on. One source of stress identified by both patients and clinicians is fear of the unknown, or not knowing what to expect. Since this is recognised as a source of stress, efforts should be made to ensure patients are given adequate information about treatment prior to starting NPWT and that effective communication is maintained between patient and clinician.

Although some studies have measured quality of life in people receiving NPWT, these studies do not tell us about patients' actual experiences. Abbotts (2010) conducted a qualitative study in order to explore patients' views of NPWT. The author adopted a 'subtle realism' theoretical basis, acknowledging the socially-constructed meanings surrounding one's external reality. Focus groups and interviews were conducted with 12 participants who had a variety of wound types, including; abdominal surgery, cardiac bypass surgery, mastectomy, toe amputation in diabetic foot, diabetic foot ulcers, skin graft over venous leg ulcer and leg degloving injury. Nine major themes emerged from the data; these were: healing, smell, embarrassment, pain, nurse training, self-care, information provision, getting out of hospital and getting back to normal. It was found that patients felt embarrassed due to the noise and aesthetics of the system and the odour of the exudate. This restricted their social life and resulted in anxieties as they worried that others would smell the exudate. Participants also reported that the nurses who cared for them were unfamiliar with the NPWT system, and that they had to demonstrate to nurses how to change dressings. A need for information regarding the system was also noted. Despite these anxieties, participants felt that the system was effective in healing their wounds.

More recently, Bolas and Holloway (2012) conducted a qualitative investigation to examine patients' experiences and perceptions of NPWT. Six participants, two male and four female, were interviewed. Two participants had wounds on their hip, two on their foot, one had an abdominal wound and one had a wound on their lower thigh/knee area. The authors adopted a phenomenological approach, allowing them to collect rich data on the patient's own experiences. Interviews covered the physical, psychological and social impact of using NPWT, lasting approximately 1 h. Three major themes were reported; an altered sense of self, new culture of technology, and restricted lives. Patients did not feel comfortable with the NPWT system as it affected their self-image through reminding them of their wound and disfigured appearance. This had a significant impact on the patient's self-esteem and motivation.

It was found that patients often felt trapped by the system due to it having to be attached to the wound. Although most patients were optimistic due to their belief that it was the most up-to-date technology, this was also a source of anxiety due to the fact that health care staff were unfamiliar with the system. Additionally, the NPWT system restricted the patient's lives on a daily basis, such as with going to the toilet and going out socially. This caused patients to feel helpless and not in control of their daily lives. Such factors could significantly impact upon patients' QoL.

In sum, NPWT appears to be an effective treatment for some patients with chronic hard to heal wounds. However, this is not to say that it is without its issues for patients. It can be bulky, noisy, restricting and socially isolating. It can cause pain and stress during certain stages of treatment and all these factors may combine to significantly impact on the patient's quality of life during the treatment regime. It is therefore important that the health care professional monitors the patient across the course of treatment to ensure that any elemental issues are clearly and promptly identified and addressed. As noted this could be before or during specific stages of treatment.

Conclusion

Treatments for wounds can bring their own issues and psychological consequences. This chapter has sought to demonstrate some of these by focussing on three different forms of treatment for chronic wounds. Although there were both similarities and differences, what is important is that the individual clinician recognises that in order for these treatments to be effective they have to be followed by the patient. If the treatment brings with it pain, stress, psychosocial issues or impacts on an individual's quality of life then patients are less likely to be concordant. It is therefore essential that treatment is monitored regularly, not just from a medical or nursing perspective but also from a psychological one. Unique and challenging difficulties associated with the individual patient undergoing specific treatments can be immediately recognised and addressed.

References

Abbade LPF, Lastoria S, Rollow HD, Stolf HO. A socio-demographic, clinical study by patients with venous ulcer. Int J Dermatol. 2005;44(12):989–92.

Abbotts J. Patients' views on topical negative pressure: 'effective but smelly'. Br J Nurs. 2010;19(20):S37–41.

Anand SC, Dean C, Nettleton R, Praburaj DV. Health-related quality of life tools for venous-ulcerated patients. Br J Nurs. 2003;12(1):48–59.

Annells M, O'Neill J, Flowers C. Compression bandaging for venous leg ulcers: the essentialness of a willing patient. J Clin Nurs. 2008;17(3):350–9. doi:10.1111/j.1365-2702.2007.01996.x.

Apostoli A, Caula C. Pain and basic functional activities in a group of patients with cutaneous wounds under VAC therapy in hospital setting (in Italian). Prof Inferm. 2008;61:158–64.

Ashby RL, et al. Clinical and cost-effectiveness of compression hosiery versus compression bandages in treatment of venous leg ulcers (Venous leg Ulcer Study IV, VenUS IV): a randomised controlled trial. Lancet. 2014;383:871–9.

Assenza M, Cozza V, Sacco E, et al. VAC (Vacuum Assisted Closure) treatment in Fournier's gangrene: personal. Clin Ter. 2011;162(1):e1–5.

Augustin M, Zschocke I, Nutzenbewertung der Ambulanten und Stationären VAC. Therapie aus Patientensicht: Multicenterstudie mit Patientenrelevanten Endpunkten [Patient evaluation of the benefit of outpatient and inpatient vacuum therapy. Multicenter study with patient-relevant end points]. MMW Fortschritte der Medizin Originalia. 2006;148(1):25–32.

Barwell JR, Taylor M, Deacon J, Davies C, Whyman MR, Poskitt KR. Ankle motility is a risk factor for healing of chronic venous Leg ulcers. Phlebology. 2001;16:38–40.

Bolas N, Holloway S. Negative pressure wound therapy: a study on patient perspectives. Br J Community Nurs. 2012;17(3):S30–5.

Briggs M, Flemming K. Living with leg ulceration: a synthesis of qualitative research. J Adv Nurs. 2007;59(4):319–28.

Briggs M, Bennett MI, Closs SJ, Cocks K. Painful leg ulceration: a prospective, longitudinal cohort study. Wound Repair Regen. 2007;15(2):186–91.

Bryan S, Dukes S. Case study: negative pressure wound therapy in an abdominal wound. Br J Nurs. 2009;18(2):S15–21.

CREST. Clinical resource efficiency support team: guidelines for the assessment and management of Leg ulceration. Belfast: CREST; 1998.

Dereure O, Vin F, Lazareth I, Bohbot S. Compression and peri-ulcer skin in outpatients' venous leg ulcers: results of a French survey. J Wound Care. 2005;14(6):265–71.

Edwards LM. Why patients do not comply with compression bandaging. Br J Nurs. 2003;12(Suppl):S5S16.

Feben K. How effective is training in compression bandaging techniques? Br J Community Nurs. 2003;8(2):80–4.

Field H. Fear of the known? District nurses practice of compression bandaging. B J Comm Nurs. 2004;(Suppl Dec):6S-15S.

Finlayson K, Edwards H, Courtney M. Factors associated with recurrence of venous leg ulcers: a survey and retrospective chart review. Int J Nurs Stud. 2009;46(8):1071–8.

Hollinworth H, Collier M. Nurses' views about pain and trauma at dressing changes: results of a national survey. J Wound Care. 2000;9(8):369–73.

Hopkins A. Ignoring lower limb oedema will lead to ineffective care. Wounds UK. 2008;4:3.

Jull A, Walker N, Hackett M, et al. Leg ulceration and perceived health: a population based case-control study. Age Ageing. 2004a;33(3):236–41.

Jull G, Kristjansson E, Dall'Alba P. Impairment in the cervical flexors: a comparison of whiplash and insidious onset neck pain patients. Man Ther. 2004b;9:89–94.

Kammerlander G, Eberlein T. Nurses' views about pain and trauma at dressing changes: a central European perspective. J Wound Care. 2002;11(2):76–9.

Karatepe O, Eken I, Acet E, et al. Vacuum assisted closure improves the quality of life in patients with diabetic foot. Acta Chir Belg. 2011;111(5):298–302.

Keskin M, Karabekmez FE, Vilmaz E. Vacuum-assisted closure of wounds and anxiety. Scand J Plast Reconstr Surg Hand Surg. 2008;42:202–5.

King B, Wesley V, Smith R. An audit of footwear for patients for patients with leg bandages. Nurs Times. 2007;103:40–3.

Kroger K, Assenheimer B. Consensus recommendation: recommendations for compression therapy for patients with venous ulcers. EWMA. 2013;13(2):41–7.

Mendonca DA, Drew PJ, Harding KG, et al. A pilot study on the effect of topical negative pressure on quality of life. J Wound Care. 2007;16(2):49–53.

Miller C, Kapp S, Newall N, et al. Predicting concordance with multilayer compression bandaging. J Wound Care. 2011;20(3):101–2, 104, 106 Passim.

Milne J. 1: Improving wellbeing of those living with a wound. Br J Nurs. 2013;22:3–9.

Moffatt MF. SPINK5: a gene for atopic dermatitis and asthma. Clin Exp Allergy. 2004a;34:325–7.

Moffatt CJ. Factors that affect concordance with compression therapy. J Wound Care. 2004b;13(7):291–6.

Moffatt C, Kommala D, Dourdin N, Choe Y. Venous leg ulcers: patient concordance with compression therapy and its impact on healing and prevention of recurrence. Int Wound J. 2009;6: 386–93.

Mudge E, Holloway S, Simmonds W, Price P. Living with venous leg ulceration: issues concerning adherence. Br J Nurs. 2006;15(21): 1166–71.

Nease C. Using low pressure, NPWT for wound preparation & the management of split-thickness skin grafts in 3 patients with complex wound. Ostomy Wound Manage. 2009;55(6):32–42.

Nelson EA. The development of a training device for users of medical compression bandages used in the treatment of chronic venous ulcers type of submission: Contributed paper type of presentation: oral presentation conference: 2012 IEEE/ASME international conference on advanced intelligent mechatronics submission number: 4. In: Conference on advanced intelligent mechatronics, Taiwan, 2012.

O'Meara S, et al. Four layer bandage compared with short stretch bandage for venous leg ulcers: systematic review and meta-analysis of randomised controlled trials with data from individual patients. BMJ. 2009;338:b1344.

Ousey K, Bianchi J, Beldon P, Young T. Identification and treatment of moisture lesions. Wounds UK (Suppl). 2012. Available from: www.wounds-uk.com.

Panicker VN. A pilot study evaluating topical negative pressure using V1STA technology. Wound Pract Res. 2009;17(4):194.

Parvaneh S, Grewal GS, Grewal E, Menzies RA, Talal TK, Armstrong DG, Sternberg E, Najafi B. Stressing the dressing: Assessing stress during wound care in real-time using wearable sensors. Wound Med. 2014;4:21–6.

Price JR, Mitchell E, Tidy E, Hunot V. Cognitive behaviour therapy for chronic fatigue syndrome in adults. Cochrane Database Syst Rev. 2008a;(3):CD0010207.

Price PE, Fagervik-Morton H, Mudge EJ, Beele H, Conteras Ruiz J, Huldt Nystrom T, Harding KG. Dressing- related pain in patients with chronic wounds: an international patient perspective. Int Wound J. 2008b;5(2):159–71.

Puffett N, Martin L, Chow MK. Cohesive short-stretch vs four-layer bandages for venous leg ulcers. Br J Community Nurs. 2006;11(6):S6, S8, S10–1.

Randell R, Mitchell N, Thompson C, McCaughan D, Dowding D. Supporting nurse decision making in primary care: exploring use of and attitude to decision tools. Health Informatics J. 2009;15(1):5–16.

Rippon M, Davies P, White R, Bosanquet N. Cost implications of using an a-traumatic dressing in the treatment of acute wounds. J Wound Care. 2008;17(5):224–7.

Royal College of Nursing. The nursing management of patients with venous leg ulcers. London: RCN; 2006.

Sadler GM, Russell GM, Boldy DP, Stacey MC. General practitioners' experiences of managing patients with chronic leg ulceration. Med J Aust. 2006;185(2):78–81.

Satpathy A, Hayes S, Dodds SR. Measuring sub-bandage pressure: comparing the use of pressure monitors and pulse oximeters. J Wound Care. 2006;15(3):125–8.

Schimp VL, Worley C, Brunello S, et al. Vacuum-assisted closure in the treatment of gynecologic oncology wound failures. Gynecol Oncol. 2003;92:586–91.

SIGN. The care of patients with chronic leg ulcer. 1998. http://www.sign.ac.uk/guidelines/index.html.

Solowiej K, Mason V, Upton D. Psychological stress and pain in wound care, part 3: management. J Wound Care. 2010a;19(4):153–5.

Solowiej K, Mason V, Upton D. Psychological stress and pain in wound care, part 2: a review of pain and stress assessment tools. J Wound Care. 2010b;19(3):110–5.

Stansby G, Wealleans V, Wilson L, Morrow D, et al. Clinical experience of a new NPWT system in diabetic foot ulcers and post-amputation wounds. J Wound Care. 2010;19(11):496.

Stephen-Haynes J. An overview of compression therapy in leg ulceration. Nurs Stand. 2006;20(32):68–76.

Templeton S, Telford K. Diagnosis and management of venous leg ulcers: a nurse's role? Wound Pract Res. 2010;18(2):72–9.

Thomas S. The use of the Laplace equation in the calculation of sub-bandage pressure. EMWA J. 2003;3(1). Available from URL: http://www.worldwidewounds.com/2003/june/Thomas/Laplace-Bandages.htm.

Todd M. Venous leg ulcers and the impact of compression bandaging. Br J Nursing. 2011;20(21):1360–4.

Todd M. Chronic oedema: impact and management. Br J Nurs. 2013; 22(11):623–7.

Ubbink DT, Westerbos SJ, Evans D, Land L, Vermeulen H. Topical negative pressure for treating chronic wounds. Cochrane Database Syst Rev. 2008;(3):CD001898.

Upton D, Andrews A. Negative pressure wound therapy: improving the patient experience, part two of three. J Wound Care. 2013a;22(11):582–91.

Upton D, Andrews A. Negative pressure wound therapy: improving the patient experience, part one of three. J Wound Care. 2013b;22(10):552–7.

Upton D, Andrews A. Pain and trauma in negative pressure wound therapy: a review. Int Wound J. 2013c; Advance online publication.

Upton D, Solowiej K. The impact of a traumatic vs conventional dressings on pain and stress. J Wound Care. 2012;21(5):209–15.

Upton D, Hender C, Solowiej K. Mood disorders in patients with acute and chronic wounds: a health professional perspective. J Wound Care. 2012a;21(1):42–8.

Upton D, Hender C, Solowiej K, Woo K. Stress and pain associated with dressing change in chronic wound patients. J Wound Care. 2012b;22(2):53–61.

Upton D, Solowiej K, Hender C, Woodyat KY. Stress and pain associated with dressing change in patients with chronic wounds. J Wound Care. 2012c;21(2):53–61.

Van Hecke AV, Mundy P, Acra F, Block J, Delgado CEF, Parlade MV, et al. Infant joint attention, temperament, and social competence in preschool children. Child Dev. 2007;78(1):53–69.

Verbelen J, Hoeksema H, Heyneman A, Pirayesh A, Monstrey S. Treatment of Fournier's gangrene with a novel negative pressure wound therapy system. Wounds. 2011;23(11):342–9.

Wallin AM, Bostrom L, Ulfvarson J, Ottoson MD. Negative pressure wound therapy: a descriptive study. Ostomy Wound Manage. 2011;57(6):22–9.

Weller CD, Buchbinder R, Johnston RV. Interventions for helping people adhere to compression treatments for venous leg ulceration. Cochrane Database Syst Rev. 2013;(9):CD008378.

White R. A multinational survey of the assessment of pain when removing dressings. Wounds UK. 2008;4(1):1–6.

Wolvos T. Wound instillation – the next step in negative pressure wound therapy. Lessons learned from initial experiences. Ostomy Wound Manage. 2004;50(11):56–66.

World Union of Wound Healing Societies. Principles of best practice: wound exudate and the role of dressings. A consensus document. London: MEP; 2007.

Chapter 7
Concordance

> Box 7.1: Key Points
> - Concordance has been suggested to be the 'single most important modifiable factor that compromises treatment outcome' (WHO 2003);
> - Non-concordance rates in chronic wounds is around 50 %;
> - Compliance and adherence are alternative labels for patient behaviour in regard to prescribed treatment, however these have lost favour in recent years because of the paternalistic view of medicine which they embody;
> - Ley's Cognitive Hypothesis Model (1989) suggests that patient understanding and recall of information provided during a consultation, and satisfaction with their care, will influence patient treatment concordance;
> - Other factors that impact on concordance include a patient's health beliefs, illness perceptions, and social support;
> - Using a patient centred approach, which takes a patient's beliefs, lifestyle and needs into account when developing a treatment plan has been advocated to enhance concordance;
> - The patient-clinician relationship is therefore central: clear communication within a therapeutic, non-judgmental relationship appears to hold the key to good concordance.

Summary

Different terms have been used to describe patient behaviour when advised by a practitioner to take medication or make significant changes to their lifestyle. Compliance refers to the patient following the practitioner's orders obediently without question, whilst adherence implies that the patient follows the request with more negotiation. More recently the term concordance has been used to describe treatment related behaviour, particularly in the UK. Concordance implies a complete power balance between the clinician and the patient in which they work on equal terms to reach an agreement regarding treatment. Rates of non-concordance vary, depending on the nature and duration of the illness as well as a number of patient variables. However, non-concordance in chronic wounds is similar to other chronic illnesses, standing at around 50 %. According to Ley's (1989) cognitive hypothesis model, concordance is predicted by the patient's understanding of the information provided during the consultation, how well they can recall this information, and overall satisfaction with the consultation. The way information is communicated can have an impact on the way the patient recalls and understands what has been communicated. To ensure that information is communicated effectively it should be clear, simple and jargon free. Furthermore, using more than one mode of communication will enhance patient recall (for example using written as well as spoken information). A patient's health beliefs and perceptions about the causes and consequences of their wound may also influence treatment concordance. In addition social support can also have a positive influence on concordance, however the most effective support seems to be that provided by family and peers. The clinician can also provide social support to the patient, however, the most successful type is informative or educational support. Finally, there is an important link between patient-centred consultations and good concordance; clear communication within a therapeutic, non-judgmental relationship appears to hold the key to good concordance (see Box 7.1).

Introduction

Optimum outcomes in wound care are only possible with effective treatments that are implemented meticulously. According to the World Health Organisation, patient concordance is the 'single most important modifiable factor that compromises treatment outcome' (WHO 2003). Good concordance can therefore have an important influence in preventing relapse and optimising health care (Wahl et al. 2005). In contrast, non-concordance with prescribed treatments has implications for the health of the patient, the effective use of resources, and the assessment of the clinical effectiveness of treatments (Playle and Keeley 1998). Indeed, the implications for the patient of non-concordance to prescribed treatment range from an increase of symptoms and deterioration of health, through compromised quality of life, to a potential risk to life (WHO 2003); the potentially serious impact which poor concordance can have for a patient with a wound has been noted (Hallett et al. 2000).

Up to 80 % of patients can be expected not to comply with their treatment at some time (Dunbar-Jacob et al. 1995), and patients with chronic health problems tend to have the highest non-concordance rates for treatment and lifestyle changes. This is because risk of poor concordance increases with the duration and complexity of treatment regimes, and both long duration and complex treatment are characteristic of chronic health problems such as wounds. Non-concordance rates are thought to average 50 % for long-term health conditions (WHO 2003), with similar figures being reported for a range of chronic wound types (e.g. Ertl 1992; Erickson et al. 1995; Stewart et al. 2000).

It has been suggested that concordance can be either intentional or unintentional. However, explanations for non-concordance differ depending on the respondent's viewpoint. In a comprehensive review of the literature concerning concordance in patients with leg ulcers, Van Hecke et al. (2008) found that nurses focused primarily on patient-related factors such as poor motivation, lack of understanding and unwillingness to follow the treatment regime. In addition, nurses stated that patients might deliberately ignore the treatment instructions they had been given in an attempt to delay wound healing so as to prolong nursing visits (although limited evidence on this viewpoint is available- see Chap. 8). However, this tendency to see patients as being at fault when treatment plans are not followed correctly has been criticized for lacking the 'spirit of co-operation' necessary for good concordance (Kyngäs et al. 2000). In contrast, the patients themselves mentioned pain and discomfort as the main reasons for not following treatment instructions, suggesting a very different perspective on why treatment protocols were discarded. The development of a therapeutic, non-judgmental relationship would have allowed those patients to express their concerns about the suggested treatment in an open and honest way (Furlong 2001; Moffatt 2004a, b), which would allow the negotiation (by patient and clinician) of a more acceptable treatment plan resulting in better concordance.

Thus a number of factors are though to influence patient concordance and these are discussed in detail in this chapter. In particular, the role of the clinician, and the importance of good communication in enabling patient concordance with medical advice and prescribed treatment is key; the implications of this for the consultation process are therefore explored fully and recommendations for facilitation of patient concordance with wound care are provided. However, it is important to start this discussion by defining what is meant by the term concordance, and two closely related terms that are also used in the literature – compliance and adherence.

Defining the Terms Compliance, Adherence and Concordance

The terms compliance, adherence and concordance have all been used to refer to the extent to which a patient follows treatment protocols. Sometimes they are used interchangeably, however whilst these terms are related, they are not synonyms and each has a very specific meaning. Compliance was the term used during early work that investigated whether or not patients followed their practitioner's instructions. Compliance has been defined as 'the extent to which the patient's behaviour matches the prescriber's recommendations' (Horne et al. 2005). The term compliance implies that the patient will follow the clinicians orders without any question; its use is therefore declining because of an implied lack of patient involvement.

Indeed, the term compliance has been heavily criticised in the literature for its paternalistic view of the practitioner–patient relationship, in which the patient is perceived as passive and expected to obey the clinician's orders (Snelgrove 2006). Many clinicians feel uneasy about the use of the label compliance, as it places all blame for departures from prescribed treatment on the patient (Russell et al. 2003). For example, labelling the patient as non-compliant, suggests deliberate, deviant behaviour. Thus the term compliance does not allow the clinician to distinguish between patients who have intentionally decided not to take medication and those who have perhaps misunderstood what the treatment requires and as a result have not followed the prescribed treatment correctly. It has therefore been argued that the notion of compliance fails to take sufficient account of the social context of patients' lives (Russell et al. 2003) and the patient perspective on treatment (Snelgrove 2006).

This shift in perspective regarding compliance is part of a much broader change in models of patient care (DOH 2010; Coulter and Collins 2011). Thus in the past 20 or so years there has been an increasing move from clinician–patient consultations which are heavily dominated by the practitioner, who instructs the patient in 'what to do', to consultations which are more patient-centred. Patient (or person) centred care is a model of care in which patients are seen as equal partners in the planning and evaluation of their care, in order to ensure they have the most appropriate treatment plan for their needs. As a result, there is more emphasis on patients being encouraged to ask questions and the consultation focusing on a patient's individual needs. The term adherence has been used to reflect this shift in thinking.

Adherence is defined as 'the extent to which the patient's behaviour matches agreed recommendations from the prescriber' (Horne et al. 2005). The use of the phrase 'agreed recommendations' moves away from the idea of the patient as a passive recipient of health care who needs to obey the directions given by all-knowing professionals; adherence implies greater patient commitment to treatment, introduces an element of reasonable negotiation, and reflects increased patient empowerment.

The term adherence has, however, been criticised for not moving far enough away from traditional paternalistic models of care. Snelgrove (2006) suggests that whilst the reference to adherence acknowledges the negotiation between patient and clinician, it still suggests a certain degree of patient passivity, and implies that the power in the relationship remains predominantly with the clinician. In a response to this, some clinicians and researchers have used the term concordance in place of either compliance or adherence. The advantage of this term is that it suggests that the patient is an equal partner, one who shares in the decision-making process (Weiss and Britten 2003). Metcalfe (2005) succinctly summarises the similarity between compliance and adherence and their difference to concordance noting that whilst compliance and adherence can refer to behaviour by one person, concordance cannot – by definition concordance requires an active discussion, and therefore involves more than one individual. The idea of patient concordance is very much in line with the current ethos in modern heath care which puts a high value patient autonomy, self-regulation and self-management, particularly in relation to long-term conditions and chronic illness. The emphasis is on shared decision making, which takes into account a patient's circumstances, wants and desires. Concordance also demands that the clinician focuses on the consultation process, ensuring they adapt it to suit the needs of the individual patient (Metcalfe 2005).

There has however, been some criticism of concordance as a concept and the terms adherence and compliance continue to be used in preference by some clinicians and researchers. Segal (2007) for example, has suggested that the use of the term concordance is a sham, and that this new focus on joint decision making has not made any difference to the extent to which patients follow prescribed treatments. Indeed Segal (2007) goes further, suggesting that concordance is simply compliance by another name. She argues that clinicians use this concept as a guide for asking how best to persuade patients to do as they say, rather than for asking how they can ensure they demonstrate respect for the patient perspective. Whilst it is true that the need for concordance puts emphasis on the communication between clinician and patient, this should not be about the power of persuasion. Communication, as discussed throughout this chapter, is about listening as well as talking. As Metcalfe (2005) notes, there will always be some determined patients who will choose their own course of action even in the face of good evidence which contradicts said action. In these cases, the clinician should make their opinion and advice clear, but may have to accept they can do no more. Likewise at the other extreme, there will be patients that simply want to be directed by their clinician – in these instances clear communication will still be essential, and if that is the patient standpoint, such an approach remains concordant. However, for those patients (the majority) who do want to engage in meaningful discussion about their treatment plan, involving them in planning and decision making is essential; for these patients, simply telling them what they must do is likely to be counter-productive (Metcalfe 2005).

Models of Concordance

Various models have tried to explain why patients choose to follow medical advice. The most enduring of these is the Cognitive Hypothesis Model (Fig. 7.1) developed by Phillip Ley (1981, 1989). According to this model, the extent to which a patient follows prescribed treatment can be predicted by:

- their understanding of the information provided during the consultation;
- their recall of this information;
- their satisfaction with the process of the consultation

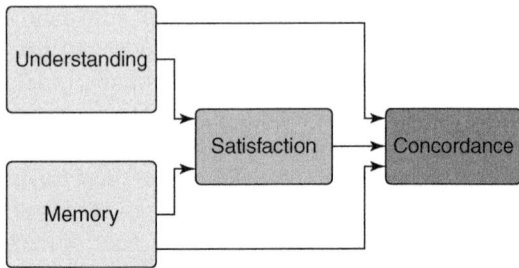

Figure 7.1 Ley's cognitive hypothesis model (Adapted from Ley (1981))

This perspective explains concordance by focusing on the communication between clinician and patient, with the most important part of this communication concerning the transfer of knowledge from expert to layperson. According to Ley's model, concordance will depend on both the clinician's skill as a communicator and the cognitive skills of the patient. Poor concordance is therefore often a product of failure to understand or recall instructions and advice, rather than a deliberate strategy of avoidance. Indeed, research from wound care practice has highlighted lack of patient understanding as one reason for poor concordance (e.g. Flanagan et al. 2001; Hallett et al. 2000). Furthermore, studies have shown that:

- Patients forget much of what the doctor tells them – according to Kessels (2003) 40–80 % of the medical information clinicians offer is forgotten immediately;
- Instruction and advice are forgotten more readily than other kinds of information (Kessels 2003);
- The more patient is told, the lower the proportion correctly recalled (McGuire 1996);
- Patients remember what they are told first and what they think is most important – information about diagnosis for example tends to be viewed as more important than information related to treatment (Kessels 2003).

According to Kessels (2003) there are three factors which can influence how likely a patient is to forget treatment instructions. The first of these relates to the mode of communication which is used. For example, if patients are provided with both oral and written information, the more likely they are to remember to follow those instructions (McDonald et al. 2002). This is because information that is received by more than one sense is more likely to be registered within memory and retained for a longer period of time. Furthermore, the written instructions will act as a memory aid, a resource which can be returned to as and when necessary. Written instructions do however present difficulties to patients with literacy problems and other options to support the oral information provided by a clinician have therefore been explored. One method which seems to be beneficial for patients with low education is the use of illustration. For example, cartoons have been used to improve patient concordance with wound-care advice after treatment in an emergency department. Those patients who received the cartoon instructions showed better understanding of what was required of them and better concordance (Delp and Jones 1996).

The second factor which may increase patient forgetfulness and so decrease concordance also concerns communication. This time however, the focus is on the behaviour of the clinician – for example the over use of medical jargon. There is substantial evidence that ineffective communication between patients and health care providers is a major determinant of poor treatment concordance (Levinson and Chaumeton 1999). Furthermore, communication is often the aspect of care with which patients are least satisfied (Aharony and Strasser 1993). For example, Stewart et al. (2000) found that 44 % of the burns patients he interviewed reported not understanding the instructions they were given in the use of pressure garments; 90 % of their consultants, however, believed the instructions were clear and the patients had understood. It is suggested that the personal backgrounds of health care providers and the norms, beliefs, and practices intrinsic to their professional training, affect their communication and interaction with patients, which ultimately affects the treatment they provide (Bates et al. 1997).

Finally Kessels notes that there are features specific to each patient which can impact on what a patient remembers about treatment needs. This includes factors such as low education that, as noted earlier, can limit a patient's understanding of instructions. It also includes a patient's own expectations of the consultation process, and their beliefs about health and healing. Indeed, individual factors such as this have been found to be very important in determining patient concordance (Snelgrove 2006). Ley's model has been criticised for not taking the possible influence of patients' pre-existing knowledge and beliefs, or life context, into account. Thus whilst Ley's model is important because of it focuses on the dialogue between patient and health care provider, it has been argued that it is an educational model, which assumes that the clinician is the expert and the patient is a novice who needs to be taught what to do (Snelgrove 2006). Any consideration of concordance however, must recognise issues such as a patient's health beliefs, their personal circumstances including social support, and their sense of control, as these are all factors which have been shown to affect the extent to which patient's will follow a treatment plan (Stanton 1987).

Health Beliefs, Self-Regulation and Illness Perception

Concordance acknowledges that whilst the health beliefs of the patient may be different to those of their clinician, they are just as relevant when making treatment choices (Dickinson et al. 1999). This is important, since the extent to which someone will engage in a health related behaviour (e.g. wound treatment) depends upon the value they put on the goal of the behaviour (e.g. wound healing) and their estimate of the likelihood that the behaviour will achieve that goal (Janz and Becker 1984). Thus according to the health belief model (HBM) (Janz and Becker 1984; Rosenstock et al. 1988) concordance with treatment will occur when a patient is:

1. Sufficiently concerned about their wound;
2. Feels threatened by the medical and social consequences of leaving the wound untreated;
3. Believes that the recommended treatment will reduce the medical and social consequences of the wound and that these benefits outweigh the costs of engaging in the treatment;
4. Believes that they can successfully carry out the prescribed treatment (self-efficacy)

According to the HBM, by weighing up the pros and cons of taking therapeutic action such as wearing compression bandages, people arrive at a decision as to whether the perceived benefits (e.g. wound healing, or prevention of recurrence) outweigh the perceived barriers or cost (e.g. Compression causing pain and discomfort at night; Crookes 1997). As Moffatt (2004a, b) notes, it is important to understand the patient's beliefs about compression during consultation, particularly if there have been previous episodes of failed treatment. Research into the extent to which burns patients wear the pressure garments which they are prescribed also supports the HBM; Stewart et al. (2000) found that 56 % of burns patients were uncertain about the ability of their pressure garments to reduce their hypertrophic scars with almost a third of the sample not wearing the pressure garments they had been prescribed for the full 20–24 h that were recommended.

Self-care can be an important part of wound management, as it was for the burns patients in the study by Stewart and colleagues (2000). One of the barriers to wearing the pressure suit which was described by patients, concerned the difficulty of putting on and taking off the garment they had been prescribed. Another barrier related to the challenge of coping with the itching and discomfort created by the suit. Those patients who described difficulties donning and wearing the suit could be said to lack self-efficacy – that is the belief that they can cope with, or carry out particular behaviours. Patients who felt unable to cope with the discomfort would be less likely to wear their suit for the recommended length of time; those finding it difficult to get the garment on and off might stop wearing it all together. Self-efficacy therefore has important implications for concordance in cases where self-care is required. Low levels of self-efficacy have been also been implicated in patients with leg ulcers who do not engage in physical exercise (Heinen et al. 2007), poor concordance with compression bandaging (Finlayson et al. 2010), and poor foot-care in people with diabetic neuropathic foot complications (Vileikyte et al. 2004).

Patient beliefs are also central to the self-regulatory theory or 'common sense' model of illness, put forward by Leventhal and colleagues (Leventhal and Cameron 1987; Leventhal et al. 1997, 2003). According to this model, 'common-sense' beliefs about illness and their remedies shape our response to threats to our health. Thus we expect aspirin to cure a headache, antibiotics to clear infection, ointment to soothe an itchy rash and so on (Leventhal et al. 2003). When our expectations are fulfilled (e.g. the ointment soothes the itch), behaviours are reinforced and we are more likely to repeat them in the future. However, if our expectations are thwarted then we will reassess the situation, questioning the relevance of the remedy (perhaps this rash is more serious than first imagined) or its efficacy. Concordance behaviours are therefore heavily influenced by these common-sense beliefs, and the patient's 'illness perceptions', that is their representations of their illness. Illness perceptions differ from person to person (Cameron and Leventhal 2003) and even patients with the same medical condition can hold very disparate views of their illness. The way that patients think about their illness is structured around five cognitive dimensions:

1. **illness identity** – the label an individual gives to their illness and the symptoms that they believe are associated with the condition;
2. **timeline** – how long the patient expects the condition to last;
3. **causes** of the illness;
4. **consequences** of their health problem;
5. **control** over disease progress (can treatment effect a cure)

According to this model, concordance is regulated by the patient, who monitors their treatment in light of these five attributes. For example, a patient with a leg ulcer whose **illness identity** includes symptoms such as pain, exudate and malodour will monitor the use of compression bandages, evaluating how this affects these symptoms. If the desired effect – reduced pain, exudate and malodour – is realized in the **timeline** the patient anticipates, so reducing the **consequences** of the ulcer (e.g. reduced mobility, embarrassment) they will maintain treatment behaviour because they believe the treatment is effective and has given them **control** over illness progression. If these symptoms do not reduce, then the patient may, for example, begin to doubt the efficacy of the prescribed intervention (Charles 1995) and stop engaging in treatment behaviours. As Moffatt (2004a, b) notes, a patient's previous experience with wound care therapies will impact on their attitudes towards, and beliefs about those therapies and their subsequent concordance.

Patients' beliefs about their condition and aims for treatment re often at variance from those who are treating them; for example, clinicians may see healing as the priority, whilst the patient's priority might be to reduce pain and feel comfortable (Morgan and Moffatt 2008). Likewise it has been demonstrated that patients frequently fail to understand the underlying cause of their wound and that until this is tackled healing will not take place (Edwards et al. 2002). Awareness of these five cognitive dimensions can help the clinician to understand how the patient makes sense of their illness and its treatment, thereby promoting a more patient centred approach to care.

Social Support

Research suggests that positive social support is very effective for boosting concordance (DiMatteo 2004). Likewise a lack of social support can reduce the likelihood of treatment concordance; for example, Stewart et al. (2000) linked high rates of non-concordance in burns patients, to a lack of encouragement from their families to wear their pressure garments. The family appears to be particularly important in this regard, with concordant patients being more likely to report at least one family member supporting them in following recommended treatment regimens (Barnhoorn and Adriaanse 1992; Liefooghe et al. 1995). According to social learning theory (Ajzen and Fishbein 1980), patients are much more likely to engage in health-promoting behaviour when their significant others have high expectations that the patient will engage in that behaviour as opposed to when such expectations are lacking; the expectations and encouragement of others (or the imposition of sanctions for non-concordance) is likely to act as an external motivation, and as has already been discussed, patients need to be motivated to follow treatment regimes.

The importance of social support is very significant for wounds patients; as already noted in Chap. 2, a number of physical and psychosocial factors associated with having a wound may lead to social isolation in these patients (and the importance of social support is detailed in Chap. 8). For these, and others patients (such as the elderly) who may not have family or friends living very close to them, the immediate social support network may be the clinician. Furthermore, the social support provided by clinicians has been shown to promote adherence in some patients (Sherbourne et al. 1992). There are a number of different kinds of social support from emotional through to educational/informational support (Heaney and Israel 2002). Whilst the clinician can provide different kinds of social support to the patient, there is evidence that the most effective support from the health care practitioner is informational (Heaney and Israel 2002) – so providing information about the wound and its healing, providing instructions to the patient about interventions and treatment. It has however been suggested that patients do not see nurses as social support contacts (Charles 2010) and that patients need emotional support from family and friends rather than from health care professionals (Blanchard et al. 1995). This may be in part because of the power differential between the health care professional and the patient and this has led to interventions in which recovered patients are recruited and trained to provide social support as lay health advisors (e.g. Berkman et al. 2000; Freidman et al. 2006). An alternative method of tapping into the expertise of patients is to develop self-help groups (Heaney and Israel 2002). A good example of this approach is provided by the Lindsay leg clubs (Lindsay 2001) which is discussed in more detail in Chap. 8. In this model, community-based leg ulcer care is provided to patients in a non-medical social setting such as a local village hall. The emphasis is on social interaction, the sharing of experiences and peer support. Evidence has shown a positive impact on patient concordance; in a study of 93 leg club attendees, Lindsay (2001) found a marked improvement in concordance from 17 to 5 % over an 11 month period.

The mechanism by which social support promotes concordance is likely to be very complex. Support from family and friends can be both direct -changing patient behaviours, and giving practical assistance – and indirect – encouraging optimism, increasing self-esteem, acting as a buffer for the stress of being ill, reducing patient depression (DiMatteo 2004). However, the exact means by which social support contributes to concordance is not yet completely understood. The impact of significant others on treatment concordance may be purely behavioral, or it may be physiological, impacting on mechanisms such as immune system and endocrine functioning (Druley and Townsend 1998). Alternatively social support may work indirectly by increasing another factor known to influence concordance – patient satisfaction with medical care (Da Costa et al. 1999).

Patient Satisfaction and Patient Centred Care

Patient satisfaction is thought to be one of the major contributing factors to concordance. In particular, it is argued that the extent to which health care providers are able to identify the specific needs of their patients for information, support, and reinforcement (Hill 1989) is directly related to the level of satisfaction with health care (Vojnovic et al. 1997) and to the future trajectory of their health outcomes (Mechanic 1992). Communication during the consultation is therefore of prime importance for determining patient satisfaction.

Wolf et al. (1978, 1981) measured specific parts of a consultation, to determine what actually resulted in patient satisfaction. Wolf and his colleagues found that there were four specific aspects of the consultation that appeared to be instrumental in influencing patient satisfaction, three of which related specifically to the communication process:

- satisfaction with treatment
- communication comfort – satisfaction with the doctors' ability to make it easy to talk about their problems
- rapport – satisfaction with the warmth and friendliness in the atmosphere during the consultation
- distress relief – satisfaction with the doctors' ability to relieve the patients of their worries

Whilst Wolf's study concerned consultations by medics, the evidence suggests that patient satisfaction focuses on the same elements whether the consultation is carried out by a medic or another health care professional such as a nurse (Poulton 1996). Like Wolf, Poulton also found that patient satisfaction was related to feeling they could confide in the clinician, feeling listened to and understood, improved understanding of their illness and its treatment.

It seems therefore that patients are more satisfied with health care when the consultation is patient-centred (Little et al. 2001) – that is it focuses on them as an individual, not just their illness (Mallinger et al. 2005) and this is an approach that has been advocated widely in wound care (Reddy et al. 2003a, b; Bale and Jones 2006; Van Rijswijk and Gray 2012). Furthermore there is well documented evidence that the patient centred approach is a highly effective way of increasing concordance (Lindsay 2000). Patient centred care has been described and defined in a number of different ways, however there are three key features of a patient centred consultation:

- the clinician's ability to elicit the patient's concerns;
- the consideration of the patients' psychosocial needs;

- the involvement of the patient in decisions about treatment.

The patient will therefore be more satisfied and less anxious if they feel that they have been understood and their requests have been met (Like and Zyzanski 1986, 1987). This in turn will lead to better concordance (Kerse et al. 2004). To ensure that the patient has had all their questions answered satisfactorily, and any misunderstandings clarified, the clinician will have to bear in mind that the patient might be viewing their illness and its treatment through a different lens to the clinician due to their individual heath beliefs and illness perceptions.

To ensure a patient centred consultation, clinicians will also need to evaluate the extent to which the patient wishes to be involved in decision-making (McKinstry 2000). Whilst there is some evidence that the majority of patients do want healthcare practitioners to take a patient centred approach (Little et al. 2001), there is also evidence that the aspect of patient centred care that is universally valued concerns communication. In contrast the desire for involvement in treatment decisions depends on a number of different factors including the patient's age, sex and social background, and the type and duration of illness (McKinstry 2000). Thus there is a tendency for males, older patients, those from a lower socio-economic background and with a lower level of education to prefer clinicians to take a more directive approach, although these associations are not absolute, with large minorities in each group (McKinstry 2000). However, evidence does support the desirability of shared decision-making in chronic illness (McKinstry 2000; Joosten et al. 2008). Not only does shared decision making appear to be more desired in long term conditions, it also appears that it may be more effective for concordance (Joosten et al. 2008). It has therefore been suggested that clinicians need to take a flexible approach to patient-centred consultation in order to enhance patient satisfaction and concordance (Swenson et al. 2004). Clinicians therefore need the skills, to determine when and to what extent their patients wish to be involved in decision making in order to be truly patient centred.

Implications for Practice

Concordance relies to a great extent on patient satisfaction with the consultation process, thus in order to achieve good concordance it is necessary to develop a therapeutic, non-judgmental relationship with patients living with a wound (Moffatt 2004a, b). As a part of this process the clinician needs to ensure they:

- Understand the patient's attitudes, knowledge and beliefs about their illness, its causes and consequences;
- Understand the patient's lifestyle, and how treatment will be fitted into this, discussing any modifications that might be necessary – either to lifestyle or treatment regime;
- Understand the patient's beliefs about the recommended treatment protocol, which includes being aware of any previous episodes of failed treatment that might impact on the patient's expectations;
- Identify the degree to which the patient wishes to be involved in their care, including the adoption of self-care treatment plans;
- Engage the patient in decision making about the choice of treatment if they wish to be involved in this process;
- Undertake assessment of the psychosocial factors that can affect concordance including pain, stress, depression and social support and include this knowledge in treatment planning;
- Communicate clearly, keeping information as simple (but accurate) as possible and avoid the use of jargon;
- Discuss the most important instructions and information at the beginning of the consultation;
- Provide any information or instructions in more than one medium, choosing those that are most appropriate for the patient's knowledge and skills (e.g. written and spoken, pictorial and spoken);
- Monitor the patient's understanding of, and concordance with the agreed treatment regime by asking questions to ensure recall is accurate;
- Provide prompts and reminders about treatment and encourage self-monitoring of progress.

Consultation with patients should not be viewed as a one off, but rather an on-going dialogue. Furthermore, it is important to remember that the more complex a regimen is, the more likely it is a patient will not show full concordance (Bender 2002), thus it is vital that a complex treatment regime is discussed and planned in light of what the patient does on a daily basis (McDonald et al. 2002). Moreover, the clinician must bear in mind that whilst a patient may show concordance with one set of treatment recommendations, they may well refuse to engage with another. However, interactions with patients should not be treated as opportunities to reinforce treatment instruction, but rather as a time for heath care professionals and patients to share their knowledge and experience of wounds and their care, in order to reach a joint treatment plan (Bissell et al. 2004). Finally, the clinician should remember that it is beholden upon them to maintain their own concordance with a treatment plan; Goreki et al. (2009) identified a dissonance between the needs of patients with a pressure ulcer and clinical and nursing needs, which led to patients feeling their needs were less important and that they were being a nuisance when asking for assistance. In contrast however, if health care professionals were able to agree symptoms and treatment plans though joint decision making with patients, providing clear communication about treatments this allowed the patient to feel in control, which ultimately led to better concordance.

Conclusion

This chapter has discussed the different factors that contribute to concordance behaviours. These include characteristics of the patient, such as health beliefs, illness perceptions and previous treatment experiences. However, through good communication during a non-judgmental consultation, a clinician who is familiar with these issues can increase the likelihood that the patient will show concordance to treatment. Thus the relationship between the clinician and the patient is probably the most important influence on the extent of patient concordance.

References

Aharony L, Strasser S. Patient satisfaction: what we know about and what we still need to explore. Med Care Rev. 1993;50(1):49–79.

Ajzen I, Fishbein M. Understanding attitudes and predicting social behaviour. Englewood Cliffs: Prentice Hall; 1980.

Bale S, Jones V. Wound care nursing: a patient-centred approach. New York: Elsevier Health Sciences; 2006.

Barnhoorn F, Adriaanse H. In search of factors responsible for non-compliance among tuberculosis patients in Wardha District, India. Soc Sci Med. 1992;34:219–306.

Bates MS, Rankin-Hill L, Sanchez-Ayendez M. The effects of the cultural context of health care on treatment of and response to chronic pain and illness. Soc Sci Med. 1997;45(9):1433–47.

Bender BG. Overcoming barriers to nonadherence in asthma treatment. J Allergy Clin Immunol. 2002;109(6):S554–9.

Berkman LF, Glass T, Brissette I, Seeman TE. From social integration to health: Durkheim in the new millennium. Soc Sci Med. 2000;51(6):843–57.

Bissell P, May CR, Noyce PR. From compliance to concordance: barriers to accomplishing a re-framed model of health care interactions. Soc Sci Med. 2004;58(4):851–62.

Blanchard CG, Albrecht TL, Ruckdeschel JC, Grant CH, Hemmick RM. The role of social support in adaptation to cancer and to survival. J Psychosoc Oncol. 1995;13(1–2):75–95.

Charles H. The impact of leg ulcers on patients' quality of life. Prof Nurse. 1995;10(9):571–3.

Charles H. The Lindsay leg club model. EWMA J. 2010;10(3):38–40.

Coulter A, Collins A. Making shared decision-making a reality. No decision about me, without me. London: King's Fund; 2011.

Crookes M. Making a fresh start. Nurs Times. 1997;93:68–74.

Da Costa D, Clarke AE, Dobkin PL, Senecal JL, Fortin PR, Danoff DS, Esdaile JM. The relationship between health status, social support and satisfaction with medical care among patients with systemic lupus erythematosus. Int J Qual Health Care. 1999;11(3):201–7.

Delp C, Jones J. Communicating information to patients: the use of cartoon illustrations to improve comprehension of instructions. Acad Emerg Med. 1996;3(3):264–70.

Department of Health. Equity and excellence: liberating the NHS. London: Stationery Office; 2010.

Dickinson D, Wilkie P, Harris M. Taking medicines: concordance is not compliance. BMJ. 1999;319(7212):787.

DiMatteo MR. Social support and patient adherence to medical treatment: a meta-analysis. Health Psychol. 2004;23(2):207.

Druley JA, Townsend AL. Self-esteem as a mediator between spousal support and depressive symptoms: a comparison of healthy individuals and individuals coping with arthritis. Health Psychol. 1998;17:255–61.

Dunbar-Jacob J, Sereika S, Rohay JM, Burke LE, Kwoh CK. Predictors of adherence: Differences by measurement method. Ann Behav Med. 1995;17:S196.

Edwards LM, et al. An exploration of patients' understanding of leg ulceration. J Wound Care. 2002;11(1):35–9.

Erickson CA, Lanza DJ, Karp DL, Edwards JW, Seabrook GR, Cambria RA, et al. Healing of venous ulcers in an ambulatory care program: the roles of chronic venous insufficiency and patient compliance. J Vasc Surg. 1995;22:629–36.

Ertl P. How do you make your treatment decision? Prof Nurse. 1992;7:543–52.

Finlayson K, Edwards H, Courtney M. The impact of psychosocial factors on adherence to compression therapy to prevent recurrence of venous leg ulcers. J Clin Nurs. 2010;29:1289–97.

Flanagan M, Rotchell L, Fletcher J, Schofield J. Community nurses', home carers' and patients' perceptions of factors affecting venous leg ulcer recurrence and management of services. J Nurs Manag. 2001;9:153–9.

Friedman LC, Kalidas M, Elledge R, Chang J, Romero C, Husain I, Dulay MF, Liscum KR. Optimism, social support and psychosocial functioning among women with breast cancer. Psychooncology. 2006;15:595–603.

Furlong W. Venous disease treatment and compliance: the nursing role. Br J Nurs. 2001;10 Suppl 2:S18–35.

Gorecki C, Brown JM, Nelson EA, Briggs M, Schoonhoven L, Dealey C, Defloor T, Nixon J & on behalf of the European Quality of Life Pressure Ulcer Project group. Impact of pressure ulcers on quality of life in older patients: a systematic review. J Am Geriatr Soc. 2009;57:1175–83.

Hallett CE, Austin L, Caress A, Luker KA. Community nurses' perceptions of patient 'compliance' in wound care: a discourse analysis. J Adv Nurs. 2000;32(1):115–23.

Heaney CA, Israel BA. Social networks and social support. In: Health behavior and health education: theory, research, and practice. 3rd ed. San Francisco: Jossey-Bass; 2002. p. 185–209.

Heinen MM, Evers AWM, Van Uden CJT, Van Der Vleuten CJM, Van De Kerkhof PCM, Van Achterberg T. Sedentary patients with venous or mixed leg ulcers: determinants of physical activity. J Adv Nurs. 2007;60(1):50–7.

Hill MN. Strategies for patient education. Clin Exp Hypertens. 1989;11(5–6):1187–201.

Horne R, Weinman J, Barber N, Elliott RA, Morgan M. Concordance, adherence and compliance in medicine taking: a conceptual map and research priorities. London: National Co-ordinating Centre for NHS Service Delivery and Organisation NCCSDO; 2005.

Janz NK, Becker MH. The health belief model: a decade later. Health Educ Q. 1984;11(1):1–47.

Joosten EA, DeFuentes-Merillas L, De Weert GH, Sensky T, Van Der Staak CPF, de Jong CA. Systematic review of the effects of shared decision-making on patient satisfaction, treatment adherence and health status. Psychother Psychosom. 2008;77(4):219–26.

Kerse N, Buetow S, Mainous AG, Young G, Coster G, Arroll B. Physician-patient relationship and medication compliance: a primary care investigation. Ann Fam Med. 2004;2(5):455–61.

Kessels RP. Patients' memory for medical information. J R Soc Med. 2003;96(5):219–22.

Kyngäs H, Duffy ME, Kroll T. Conceptual analysis of compliance. J Clin Nurs. 2000;9(1):5–12.

Leventhal H, Cameron L. Behavioral theories and the problem of compliance. Patient Educ Couns. 1987;10:117–38.

Leventhal H, Benyamini Y, Brownlee S, et al. Illness representations: theoretical foundations. In: Petrie KJ, Weinman JA, editors. Perceptions of health and illness. Amsterdam: Harwood Academic; 1997. p. 19–45.

Leventhal H, Brissette I, Leventhal EA. The common-sense model of self-regulation of health and illness. In: Cameron LD, Leventhal H, editors. The self-regulation of health and illness behaviour. London: Routledge; 2003. p. 42–65.

Levinson W, Chaumeton N. Communication between surgeons and patients in routine office visits. Surgery. 1999;125(2):127–34.

Ley P. Professional non-compliance: a neglected problem. Br J Clin Psychol. 1981;20:151–4.

Ley P. Improving patients' understanding, recall, satisfaction and compliance. In: Health psychology. USA: Springer; 1989. p. 74–102.

Liefooghe R, Michaels N, Habib S, Moran MB, De Muynck A. Perceptions and social consequences of tuberculosis: A focus group study of tuberculosis patients in Sailkot, Pakistan. Soc Sci Med. 1995;41:1685–92.

Like R, Zyzanski SJ. Patient requests in family practice: a focal point for clinical negotiations. Fam Pract. 1986;3(4):216–28.

Like R, Zyzanski SJ. Patient satisfaction with the clinical encounter: social psychological determinants. Soc Sci Med. 1987;24:351.

Lindsay E. Leg clubs: A new approach to patient centred leg ulcer management. Nurs Health Sci. 2000;2(3):139–41.

Lindsay ET. Compliance with science: benefits of developing community leg clubs. Br J Nurs. 2001;10(22 Suppl):S66–74.

Little P, Everitt H, Williamson I, Warner G, Moore M, Gould C, et al. Preferences of patients for patient centred approach to consultation in primary care: observational study. BMJ. 2001;322(7284):468.

Mallinger JB, Griggs JJ, Shields CG. Patient-centered care and breast cancer survivors' satisfaction with information. Patient Educ Couns. 2005;57(3):342–9.

McDonald HP, Garg AX, Haynes RB. Interventions to enhance patient adherence to medication prescriptions: scientific review. JAMA. 2002;288(22):2868–79.

McGuire LC. Remembering what the doctor said: organization and older adults' memory for medical information. Exp Aging Res. 1996;22:403–28.

McKinstry B. Do patients wish to be involved in decision making in the consultation? A cross sectional survey with video vignettes. BMJ. 2000;321(7265):867–71.

Mechanic D. Health and illness behavior and patient-practitioner relationships. Soc Sci Med. 1992;34(12):1345–50.

Metcalfe R. Compliance, adherence, concordance–what's in a NAME? Pract Neurol. 2005;5(4):192–3.

Moffatt MF. SPINK5: a gene for atopic dermatitis and asthma. Clin Exp Allergy. 2004a;34:325–7.

Moffatt CJ. Factors that affect concordance with compression therapy. J Wound Care. 2004b;13(7):291–6.

Morgan PA, Moffatt CJ. Non healing leg ulcers and the nurse–patient relationship. Part 2: the nurse's perspective. Int Wound J. 2008;5(2):332–9.

Playle JF, Keeley P. Non-compliance and professional power. J Adv Nurs. 1998;27:304–11.

Poulton BC. Use of the consultation satisfaction questionnaire to examine patients' satisfaction with general practitioners and community nurses: reliability, replicability and discriminant validity. Br J Gen Pract. 1996;46(402):26–31.

Reddy M, Kohr R, Queen D, Keast D, Sibbald RG. Practical treatment of wound pain and trauma: a patient-centered approach. An overview. Ostomy Wound Manage. 2003a;49(4 Suppl):2–15.

Reddy M, Keast D, Fowler E, Sibbald RG. Pain in pressure ulcers. Ostomy Wound Manage. 2003b;49(4A Suppl):30–5.

Rosenstock IM, Strecher VJ, Becker MH. Social learning theory and the health belief model. Health Educ Behav. 1988;15(2):175–83.

Russell S, Daly J, Hughes E. Nurses and 'difficult' patients: negotiating non compliance. J Adv Nurs. 2003;43(3):281–7.

Segal JZ. "Compliance" to "concordance": A critical view. J Med Humanit. 2007;28(2):81–96.

Sherbourne CD, Hays RD, Ordway L, DiMatteo MR, Kravitz RL. Antecedents of adherence to medical recommendations: results from the Medical Outcomes Study. J Behav Med. 1992;15(5):447–68.

Snelgrove S. Factors contributing to poor concordance in health care. Medicine. 2006;46(1):119–29.

Stanton AL. Determinants of adherence to medical regimens by hypertensive patients. J Behav Med. 1987;10:377–94.

Stewart R, Bhagwanjee AM, Mbakaza Y, Binase T. Pressure garment adherence in adult patients with burn injuries: An analysis of patient and clinician perceptions. Am J Occup Ther. 2000;54:598–606.

Swenson SL, Buell S, Zettler P, White M, Ruston DC, Lo B. Patient-centered Communication. J Gen Intern Med. 2004;19(11):1069–79.

Van Hecke A, Grypdonck M, Defloor T. Interventions to enhance patient compliance with leg ulcer treatment: a review of the literature. J Clin Nurs. 2008;17(1):29–39.

Van Rijswijk L, Gray M. Evidence, research, and clinical practice: a patient-centered framework for progress in wound care. J Wound Ostomy Continence Nurs. 2012;39(1):35–44.

Vileikyte L, Rubin RR, Leventhal H. Psychological aspects of diabetic neuropathic foot complications: an overview. Diabetes Metab Res Rev. 2004;20(S1):S13–8.

Vojnovic M, Martinov-Cvejin M, Grujic V. Biosocial aspects of physician-patient communication in general medicine. Med Pregl. 1997;50(9–10):395–8.

Wahl C, Gregoire JP, Teo K, Beaulieu M, Labelle S, Leduc B, Montague T. Concordance, compliance and adherence in healthcare: closing gaps and improving outcomes. Healthc Q. 2005;8(1):65–70.

Weiss M, Britten N. What is concordance? Pharm J. 2003;271:493.

WHO. Adherence to long-term therapies: evidence for action. Geneva: World Health Organization; 2003.

Wolf MH, Putnam SM, James SA, Stiles WB. The medical interview satisfaction scale: development of a scale to measure patient perceptions of physician behavior. J Behav Med. 1978;1(4):391–401.

Chapter 8
Family, Friends and Social Support

> Box 8.1: Key Points
> - Social support can be defined as the emotional and practical support that individuals provide to others through their presence and behaviour;
> - Social support has a significant impact on both mortality and morbidly with a lack of support being detrimental to health;
> - Improved concordance with treatment, supporting healthy behaviours and providing emotional support are all routes through which social support can positively impact on an individual's health;
> - There is evidence that wound healing can be promoted by the presence of social support, potentially through an improvement in concordance;
> - A number of social support interventions can be implemented which may result in improved psychological well-being, concordance and potentially healing;
> - Living with a person with a wound can bring with it a number of significant consequences not least on the individual's health;
> - Both the individual with the wound and their immediate family may suffer psychologically and socially because of the wound.

Summary

The focus for most of the other chapters in this text has been on the person with the wound and the significant psychosocial problems that they may have to confront. However, in this chapter we explore the broader social situation and how this can impact on the individual with the wound and how, in turn, that patient influences it. The concept of social support is outlined, what it is, it's relationship to health and how this relationship comes about. The relevance to wound care is articulated and how this information can be used to develop social support interventions that can improve concordance, psychological well-being and subsequently wound healing. One specific form of social support- that received from the family and the spouse or partner in particular is explored in detail. Not only are the positive benefits to the individual with the wound detailed but the burden that may result from providing this support outlined. Social support is an important element in wound care and its impact should be harnessed by the health care professional to enhance wound healing and psychological well-being. However, the health care professional should also remember not to neglect the broader family who may all be placed under considerable burden and stress by the presence of an individual with a wound.

Introduction

Human beings are social animals and the presence of others can be of considerable benefit to most- improving not only their mental but also their physical health (Thoits 2011). Indeed, much psychological, medical and sociological research has explored this phenomenon of "social support" (see Box 8.1). Thoits (2010) defined social support as an 'emotional, informational, or practical assistance from significant others, such as family members, friends, or co-workers; and that support actually may be received from others or simply perceived to be available when needed'. Research has demonstrated that social support is important for maintaining positive physical and mental health (Ozbay et al. 2007). Indeed, social support has been shown to enhance psychological well-being; which may reduce the risk of unhealthy behaviours and poor physical health (Uchino 2004). For instance, patients with poor social support have high levels of anxiety and depression than those with higher levels of social support (Oddone et al. 2011). Social isolation and low levels of social support have been shown to be associated with increased morbidity and mortality (Berkman 1995; Umberson and Montez 2010).

Although the influence of social support has been recognised for many centuries, one of the first systematic studies completed in the 1970s identified that the risk of mortality was twice as high in those with fewer social ties (Berkman and Syme 1979). Indeed, some research has suggested that the effects of limited social support are more significant than the effects of obesity, smoking or hypertension (Sapolsky 2004). Furthermore, research has indicated that low social support may hinder the recovery of certain health conditions such as cardiovascular disease, atherosclerosis, cancer or cancer recovery and even slow wound healing (Ertel et al. 2009; Everson-Rose and Lewis 2005; Uchino 2006).

As well as this wound recurrences and poor healing rates have been associated with patients having limited social support (Moffatt et al. 2006), with lower levels of social support appearing to have a significant impact on the recurrence of a leg ulcer (Finlayson et al. 2011; Wissing et al. 2001). Consequently, social support may have a significant impact on patients' healing, their psychological well-being and potentially costs for health care providers. This chapter seeks to explore the influence of social support on well-being and health before moving onto the converse: how can chronic wounds and their treatment impact on family and friends of the individual patient?

What Is Social Support?

Social support can be defined as the existence of people on whom we can rely, people who let us know that they care about, value and love us, and the support they provide for us

(Sarason et al. 1983). There is a distinction between the existence of social relationships and the functions provided by these. That is, the structure would be based on 'how many friends, colleagues, or family relationships' you have and the functional aspect would refer to what these do.

Essentially you can have lots of friends but have no interaction with them which is not useful to us. Social support can come from a variety of different sources and a variety of types of support (Cohen et al. 2000), for instance, spouses, relatives, friends, neighbours, co-workers, or superiors. But it can also come from professional sources (e.g. the nurse or other health care professional) and this can help in reducing stress, thus becoming a useful and advantageous social interaction. The type and amount of social support an individual receives depends upon their social network but also on various demographic factors such as their age, sex, culture, socioeconomic status and so on.

Generally social support comes in one of five types (see Fig. 8.1).

To explore the concepts presented in Fig. 8.1 in more detail:

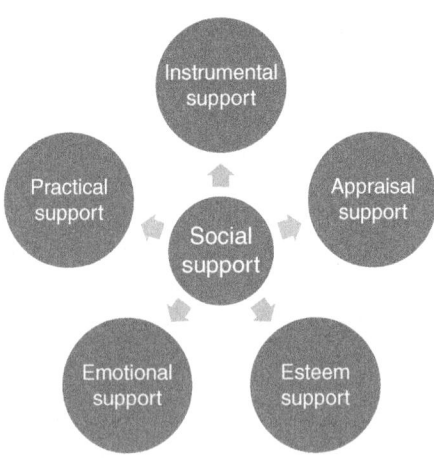

FIGURE 8.1 Sources of social support

Instrumental support: Is practical support- people will help you out when needed. They will give you a lift to the clinic, or do the shopping for you and so on.

Appraisal support: The person is encouraged to evaluate their own health through information and they are then able to put the stressors in context. In this way, the stresses and strain of the treatment is put into context and the individual realises that they are able to complete any necessary changes.

Emotional support: A "shoulder to cry on" is the traditional descriptor for this form of social support. It is being loved, cared for, protected emotionally and listened to.

Esteem support: Is a feeling that you are valued or held in esteem by others. If you feel that you are a competent and skilful person you are more likely to be able to cope with the stressors.

Information support: Is support in the form of information or knowledge which can assist the person in doing the right thing to look after themselves- providing feedback on how well they are doing, for example.

For the main part, however, social support is frequently divided into either practical support or emotional support: either "help with the shopping", or a "shoulder to cry on".

There are a number of methods available to measure social support. Phenomenological studies have investigated social support (Brown 2005a, b; Victor et al. 2002) through a formal methodological interviewing approach. Although this has a number of benefits in terms of getting to the "real data", it can be subjective and time consuming. In contrast to this interviewing technique there are a number of psychometrically developed questionnaires and scales. For example, the Social Support Questionnaire (SSQ-SF; Sarason 1986; Sarason et al. 1983, 1987). The SSQ-SF is based on two elements: the perception of the number of others available to whom a person can turn to in times of need and the degree of satisfaction with the support available. The Medical Outcomes Study:

Social Support Survey (MOS-SSS; Sherbourne and Stewart 1991) is relatively brief (12 item abbreviated version) measure of social support. It assesses four components of perceived availability of social support, including (1) Emotional support/ Informational support, (2) Tangible support (including material support), (3) Positive social interaction (does person have friends that are available to have fun), and (4) Affectionate support (including loving and nurturing relationships). The Multidimensional Scale of Perceived Social (MSPSS; Zimet et al. 1988) is another relatively brief (12 items) measure. The MSPSS assesses both the perceived availability and adequacy of emotional and instrumental social support, across the three factors relating to the source of support (i.e., Family, Friends or Significant others). The Social Provisions Scale (SPS- Russell et al. 1984) assesses six dimensions of social support received within the context of interpersonal relationships: (1) Guidance (receiving advice and/or information), (2) Reliable alliance (feeling assured that one can rely on certain others for concrete assistance if necessary), (3) Reassurance of worth (feeling important to or valued by others), (4) Opportunity for nurturance (feeling needed to provide nurturing attention to others), (5) Attachments (receiving a sense of emotional security from close relationships), and (6) Social integration (feeling a sense of belonging in a group, which includes others with similar interests). All these measures of social support demonstrate both the complexity of social support and the many facets within it.

Finally, Social support has been measured from within the family with the Family Relationship Index (FRI; Moos and Moos 1981). There are also a considerable number of psychometric measures that assess family functioning and support.

How Does Social Support Protect Health?

There is mounting evidence for the relationship between social support and psychological stress, with a lack of social support potentially increasing a patient's experiences of stress and consequently potentially affecting wound healing (Brown 2008; Solowiej and Upton 2010a, b). A number of theories have been suggested that support the link between social support, stress and its impact on wound healing.

The main effect hypothesis suggests that the more social support an individual has the better the quality of life, regardless of the person's level of stress (Helgeson 2003). In other words social support is beneficial to health and it is the absence of social support that is stressful. The more social support you have the better because large social networks provide people with regular positive experiences in terms of both emotional as well as physical support. Hence, social support promotes healthier behaviours such as exercise, eating healthily and not smoking, as well as greater adherence to medical regimes.

The buffer hypothesis proposes that social support buffers the individual against the stressor. Rather than protect a person all the time against the minor hassles and stresses of everyday life, the buffer acts when it is needed most. For example, when a person with considerable social support has a diagnosis of an illness then they *appraise* it as less stressful because they know people to whom they can turn. In contrast, those with lower social support might be unable to turn to anyone (Cohen et al. 2000). In this way an individual's social support network, such as friends and family, act as a defence against the negative impacts of stress, which, in turn, can improve wellbeing and consequently the healing of the wound (Solowiej and Upton 2010a, b; Brown 2008). Indeed, Brown (2008) suggests that aftercare to prevent social isolation and potential recurrence of the wound is important.

The social comparison theory suggests that individuals may evaluate their attitudes, beliefs and their abilities against those who are in a similar situation to them. Thus, for example, individuals with a leg wound are much more likely to compare themselves to others with a leg wound in a similar situation. Individuals may either have an upwards or downward social comparison. Those with an upward social comparison can improve the view of themselves, and create a positive perception (e.g. an individual may think that someone else wound may be close to healing and that their wound is similar to theirs). Whereas a downward social comparison occurs when an individual dissociate themselves with others who they consider to be worse off than themselves to make them feel better (e.g. an individual thinking that their wound situation is better than someone else's wound).

Uchino (2006) outlined a more detailed model that demonstrated the potential pathways between social support and health. One pathway involves behavioral processes including health behaviors and adherence to medical regimens as outlined by social control and social identity theorists (Lewis and Rook 1999 ; Umberson 1987). It is suggested that social support is health-promoting because it facilitates healthier including better adherence to medical regimes.

The other major pathway involves psychological processes that are linked to appraisals, emotions or moods (e.g., depression), and feelings of control (Cohen 1988; Gore 1981; Lin 1986). A variable that has been investigated thoroughly is **control** – defined as the extent to which a person feels they are able to change their own circumstances. Broadly, the results suggest that the more control you have the less stressful it is (e.g. Troup and Dewe 2002; Gibbons et al. 2011). Obviously, there comes a point where you have more control but also considerable responsibility and this can be stressful as well. This has important considerations when exploring self-management by the patient with the wound. It is obviously important for the health care practitioner to ensure the patient is fully involved in their own wound management and takes control over his or her own condition and treatment. However, this needs to be balanced within the confines of the patient's ability and circumstances. Responsibility and control without the ability to control leads to increased stress and all the consequences that result.

Finally, it is important for the health care professional to understand how the patient copes with their wound related problems. If the patient uses social support strategies, it may be useful to involve family and friends in their treatment. If a patient prefers a more active approach it may be useful for the patient to be given more information and become more involved with their treatments. In some cases patients may avoid dealing with their wound situation, in this case it may be helpful for the health care professional to help the patient face the facts that their wound needs treatment to heal (Vermeiden et al. 2009). It is important that health care professionals strengthen patients coping strategies as this may reduce stress and potentially improve healing.

The Impact of Social Support on Health

Living with a leg ulcer can have a detrimental impact on an individual's daily life (see Chap. 1), which can leave the patient with feelings of being trapped, living a socially restricted life, and on the whole generally feeling socially isolated (Jones et al. 2008a; Parker et al. 2012). Indeed, patients can suffer from extreme social isolation as a consequence of their wound, and this has been linked to a number of factors both psychosocial and medical: including, malodour, lack of mobility, exudate, altered body image, pain and worry over further injury to their leg (e.g. Persoon et al. 2004; Parker et al. 2012; Herber et al. 2007). Furthermore, it has been suggested that patients with chronic leg ulcers often feel as if are not fully part of society because of poor mobility, and a lack of empathy and peer support from others in their local community (Brown 2005a, b; Maida et al. 2009). Similarly, researchers have suggested that an individual may be embarrassed due to exudate and malodour, which others may perceive as poor hygiene, all of which can result in further social isolation and consequently reduced social support (Douglas 2001; Hopkins 2004a). Overall, this has negative consequences for the individual- including less socialising, which reduces the number of social contacts they may have, which again results in further isolation and a lack of social support.

Research has shown that supportive social relationships can improve health and psychological well-being. This relationship can just be one friend- as long as it is a close and supportive friendship- or a large series of good supportive relationships. Holt-Lunstad et al. (2010) reported that people who were less socially integrated had higher mortality rates. Studies have suggested that those with low levels of social support have higher mortality rates – from cardiovascular disease (e.g. Brummett et al. 2001; Frasure-Smith et al. 2000; Everson-Rose and Lewis 2005) or from cancer (e.g. Hibbard and Pope 1993) and infectious diseases (e.g. Lee and Rotheram-Borus 2001). Furthermore, an overview of longitudinal studies has shown a continuous increased mortality associated with a lack of social support and weak social ties (Quick et al. 1996). Subsequent studies have confirmed that reliable links exist between social support and better physical health (e.g. Uchino 2004; Holt-Lunstad et al. 2010).

In terms of wound healing a series of ground breaking studies in the 1990s and beyond have demonstrated a clear relationship between psychological stress and wound healing (e.g. Kiecolt-Glaser et al. 1995 and see Chap. 3). For example, in a classic study Kiecolt-Glaser and colleagues (1995) explored wound healing in two groups: a control group (healthy women) and a group (n = 13) of women caring for a demented relative. The assumption was that the care-givers were under more stress than the control group and this stress would delay wound healing. Wound healing was explored using a punch biopsy- a method used to create a small wound- and the time taken to heal recorded. There was a significant difference between the two groups with those care-givers taking 25 % longer (approximately a week) than the control group. These studies have been repeated on many occasions (Kiecolt-Glaser et al. 2002) and the relationship between stress and wound healing is well recognised.

In contrast to these deleterious effects of stress on wound healing a number of studies have indicated that social support can improve wound healing. However, many of these are with animal models of stress and social support (e.g. Detillion et al. 2004) and the link to relevant human studies, particularly those with chronic wounds is lacking. Charles (2010) did explore the influence of social support on leg ulcer healing. In a group of patients with venous leg ulcers they found that social support through a community nurse was not related to healing. However, although social support was assessed through a questionnaire route, social support was not enhanced or developed. Furthermore, many of the patients were socially isolated due to their leg wounds and the findings appeared to support the suggestion that a visit to an isolated individual by community nurses did not meet the clients' needs for social support, information exchange and empathy. Consequently, there may be a need for more formal social support interventions (Lindsay 2000, 2008; see next section).

Similarly, supportive social relationships have been demonstrated to be fundamental in patients adapting to illness as well as recovering from it (e.g. Keeling et al. 1996). However, not all social support is equally beneficial and it has been demonstrated that there are sometimes negative consequences of social support- dependency or the inhibition of recovery due to a lack of control and desire to take control of their own illness (e.g. Toshima et al. 1990). Indeed, some health care professionals wonder whether a proportion of patients want to keep their ulcers to maintain contact with their social support- their community nurses- for social contact and support (Brown 2003; Wise 1986; Brown 2005a, b; Moffatt et al. 2009). For instance, it has been suggested that some patients will deliberately delay their wound healing (e.g. take their bandages off after being treated the nurse) so their social contact with the district nurse can continue. However, it is not clear how many patients may do this, and needs to be further explored along with the underlying reasons and potential solutions for any significant problem identified. Furthermore, it has been reported by Charles (2010) that patients do not see nurses as social support contacts nor do they want to keep their ulcers in order to maintain this contact. Finally, it is also important to note that not all social support should be provided by nurses and other health care professionals- the support from significant others, such as family members, friends, or co-workers is also crucial for those suffering with chronic wounds and this will be subject to further discussion later in this chapter.

Social Support Interventions

Health care professionals are usually aware of the benefits of social support interventions for individuals with leg ulcers, even if they understand that the interventions themselves do not produce healing as a direct result (Brown 2010). It has been suggested that health care practitioners should encourage patients to become more involved in self-management, through such social support self-help groups to reduce both pain and the consequent stress it causes (Price et al. 2007; Moffatt et al. 2009; Brown 2010). 'Leg clubs' can provide individuals with an environment whereby those with similar problems can socialise in a supporting, information-sharing environment (Edwards et al. 2005). There have been a number of 'leg club' interventions set up within a community setting that have been developed which aim to improve an individual's well-being, some of these include, 'Lively legs' programme (Heinen et al. 2012); 'Look after your legs' support group (Freeman et al. 2007); and the 'Lindsay leg club'® (Lindsay 2013).

Furthermore, due to the isolation and depression experiences by ulceration patients, the Lindsay Leg Club model of care was established (Lindsay 2004). It is based in a non-medical setting such as a community, church or village hall, where those with leg wounds can have collective treatment and share their experiences, there is also open access, meaning that no appointment is required. Community based interventions also provide patients with information about their wound and how to care for their wound as well as a number of strategies with living with a wound and overcoming practical difficulties from health professionals and other patients who have similar wound related problems

(Edwards et al. 2005). Here, the reintegration of leg ulceration sufferers into the social domain is encouraged, whilst the clubs have also proved successful in progressing the removal of the negative stigma associated with such ulcerations. These clubs can conclude in a number of benefits for both the patient and their carer in that not only has treatment concordance been found to improve, but recurrence rates can decrease with overall positive healing outcomes (Lindsay 2004). This club care model supports the assumption that through the fostering of therapeutic relationships, patients can be empowered and encouraged to engage with their care, leading to improved healing rates and overall reduced ulceration reoccurrence. As such, is important for clinicians to incorporate such notions within their would care regime, focusing on patient involvement, communication and health promotion, in turn, enabling patients to become actively involved in their treatment regime.

Edwards et al. (2005) evaluated a pilot community-based 'leg club' with a sample of 33 patients with venous leg ulcers. Patients were randomized to two treatment conditions, which were either the community based leg club or treatment in their own homes. Data from both groups were collected at 12 weeks, finding significant improvements in healing in the community based 'leg club' condition compared to the home group. Furthermore, those who attended the community based leg club were able to share information with 'fellow sufferers', not only about their leg ulcers but their other similar health conditions. Therefore improved healing rates in the leg club setting group could include the beneficial effects of social interaction, peer support and the opportunity to share information with others who have similar conditions. However, the small sample used in this study limits the generalizability of the findings, also patients who were unable to travel, due to being too physically disabled or those who were unable to drive were excluded. Edwards et al. (2009) conducted another study to determine the 'leg clubs' effectiveness on a number of different outcomes, which included quality of life, morale, depression, self-esteem, social support, healing pain and functional abilities of those with chronic venous leg ulcers. Sixty-seven participants were referred for care in the community, these patients were randomised to either the 'Lindsay Leg Club' ® model of care or to home visits. Data was collected at baseline, 12 and 24 weeks. Results identified that those who received care under the 'Leg Club' model had significant outcome improvements in quality of life, morale, self-esteem, healing, pain and functional ability. This suggests that the 'Lindsay Leg Club' Model of care has the potential to improve the well-being of those with chronic leg ulcers.

Overall, the 'leg club' environment may encourage an improved motivation for compliance to treatment, as patients may be able to see the direct positive effects of the treatment on others attending. As well as this the sharing of information among members attending the 'leg club' of how to overcome difficulties, such as increases in exudate or malodour, may improve compliance to treatment. 'Leg clubs' have also shown to provide significant costs for health care providers, provide holistic care for patients, a forum for health promotion and education and an accessible setting for opportunistic early detection of wounds and their treatment (Lindsay 2004). Community 'Leg clubs' may also have the propensity to develop new ways to deliver evidence-based practise in partnership with patients and colleagues (Lindsay 2013).

It has been reported that when leg ulcers are treated at community based 'leg clubs' healing times appear to be reduced, and therefore suggesting that management of psychosocial factors as well as effective evidence based treatment are effective to promote successful wound healing and prevent recurrence. A small number of evaluations have been completed to determine the effectiveness of 'leg clubs', for instance. Leg Clubs provide a space for social activities and social engagement with separate areas for wound care treatment. In this way individuals can get their treatment whilst being able to communicate and interact with others.

Despite the positive case studies and small reports (e.g. Lindsay 2013; Shuter et al. 2011) there is little evidence from randomised controlled trials (RCTS)- the so called "gold standard"- of wound healing benefit from social support interventions (e.g. Weller et al. 2013). Despite this, social support community based interventions do appear to improve a number of significant factors, such as wound care concordance and well-being (Gordon et al. 2006; Harker 2000; Edwards et al. 2009).

Family Considerations

One key element of social support is the family- the partner or spouse in particular- and they have a key role to play supporting the patient. This may be physical support- providing care and management for the wound, or emotional support for the pain, stress, or any psychological problems that the patient may be experiencing. Indeed, there is some evidence that being in a relationship may improve wound healing (Kiecolt-Glaser and Newton 2001). Moffatt et al. (2006) reported that patients who live alone were significantly more likely to have leg ulceration than those living with a spouse, although this was a cross-sectional study and hence no direct causality could be determined.

The informal carer is a considerable resource for both the individual and the country. For example, it is suggested that there are over six million carers in the UK who provide unpaid care to someone who is ill, frail or disabled (Buckner and Yeandle 2011). This contribution to care accounts for £199 billion annually. This figure equates to £2.3 billion per week, £326 million per day, £13.6 million per hour or £18 473 for every carer in the UK (Buckner and Yeandle 2011). The support they provide is fundamental to the success of the individual patient in not only successfully managing their condition physically but also psychologically. Their support is central to adaptation to chronic illness.

Conversely, of course, the experience of the family member may also be of concern. Living with an individual may bring with it significant psychosocial concerns which may be detrimental to health for the partner or family member (Bennett et al. 2013). Indeed, the impact of chronic illness on the whole family can be significant and result in increased morbidity, impaired family dynamics and ultimately family break-ups, psychological morbidity and ill-health. This section will explore these two elements of the family involvement in wound care.

Family caregivers are recognised as an important component of support for individuals with chronic conditions (Spence et al. 2008). Many take on a supportive role with little or no training, yet are involved in an array of complex and challenging tasks, such as symptom assessment, as well as assisting with activities of daily living or helping with wound management (Aranda and Hayman-White 2001; Thomas et al. 2002). The ongoing and frequent nature of some of these wound-related routines requires family adaptation, and patients' success at maintaining these routines benefits from effective family support. Moreover, family members can take an active role in helping adults with chronic illness execute complex self-management tasks, make disease-related decisions, and cope with disease-related stress (Gleeson-Kreig et al. 2002). Partners or spouses are frequently involved in their partners' chronic health conditions (Ell 1996), often by seeking to promote greater adherence to treatment regimens. Spouses are uniquely positioned to notice such non-concordance, and as such, often are directly involved in monitoring and influencing many of their partners' health related behaviours (Trief et al. 2003).

In contrast to the positive support that the family and spouse/partner may provide they may experience some costs for their involvement. However, relatively little research has examined whether spouses incur any costs from involvement in their marital partners' chronic woundcare and most of the evidence comes from either other conditions or as a by-product of other research into the patient experience. For example, in a study by Upton and Andrews (2013a, b), respondents were asked to consider the level of sleep disturbance they experienced as a direct result of NPWT with their findings suggesting that NPWT treatment itself directly impacts on patients' sleep, particularly due to noise. However, it was also noted in this study that spouses also experienced sleep disturbance due to their partners' treatment. The impact of NPWT on family and carers is therefore another area which should be explored. Research on caregiving with other chronic illnesses (e.g. diabetes) suggests that providing care to an ill family member may lead to feelings of burden as a result of the chronic stress it elicits (Vitaliano et al. 2003). This burden may stem from the time and effort spouses devote to helping their partners, as well as from potential adverse effects on their psychological or physical health (e.g. Coyne and Smith 1991). Spouses' feelings of burden also could stem from the disruption of their own routines or the drains on their energy from having to monitor and seek to influence their partners' health behaviors on a daily basis (see Sales 2003).

Hopkins et al. (2006) reported on participants with a pressure ulcer who described their worries about their families, the impact of the ulcer on the families and their sense of gratitude towards them. Based on the findings from a study on carers by Baharestani (1994), they were right to be worried: pressure ulcers do have an enormous impact on spouses. Other studies exploring issues for patients in relation to their partners also found this essence of a 'sense of indebtedness' towards the carer (White and Greyner 1999).

Indeed, family caregivers in many studies report that the care they have to provide is one of the most significant issues for those with family members with chronic conditions and this burden may lead to the caregiver postponing their own needs (Manne and Zautra 1990; Rees et al. 2001; Riemsma et al. 1999; Baanders and Heijmans 2007). The effect on family caregivers across most chronic illnesses can be grouped into changes in social, economic, physical and mental status (Glasdam et al. 2010; Johansson and Fahlstršm 1993; Oehlenslaeger 1998; Soubhi et al. 2006). The burden of care is one of the main consequences for family caregivers with chronic illness. The patient's close family members may experience poor psychological well-being (depression, anxiety), decreased satisfaction in relationships, caregiver burden and poorer physical health (Glasdam et al. 2010). Similarly, often in significant cases the carer has to give up work which can lead to significant financial problems for the whole family.

Although the term "caregiver burden" has been used extensively and documented in a number of conditions such as HIV/AIDs, cancer, heart disease and dementia (e.g. Munro and Edwards 2010; Woods 1999; Aoun et al. 2005) little has been written about care-giving for those with a chronic wound. As Ousey et al. (2013) write there "is little investigation into the impact of an acute wound on the possible psychological impact this may have on patients' and carers' quality of life" (p. 3). The authors then went on to suggest that there was a need for both investigations and recommendations into how best to support both patients and carers:

> There needs to be clear guidelines developed on how health and social care practitioners can meet the needs of these patients and their caregivers. Participation and involvement of patients and caregivers in the development of these guidelines are essential to ensure that the patient and their caregivers are at the centre of care. (p. 6)

Given the fundamental role that unpaid carers play in the support of individuals with chronic conditions and the overall value to the country that this is estimated to bring it is surprising that little research exploring carer burden with those with a chronic wound has been reported. This is important for a number of reasons. Firstly, the heath of all should be a concern for the individual health care professional. There are many anecdotal reports of the carer suffering health difficulties themselves (including premature death) and this is something that all should try and avoid. Secondly, of course, individual carers provide valuable care and support and without them the psychological and physical health of the individual wound sufferer may deteriorate. Finally, of course, without this support more health care resources would be required which would lead to greater economic burden for all. A number of theoretically driven psychological support programmes may prove beneficial. For example, the development of coping strategies, social support networks or resilience training have all been shown to be of benefit for carers (e.g. McDonald and Hayes 2001; Li et al. 2012).

Obviously, it has to be remembered that in any caregiving situation it is not just about the burden of care. Buckner and Yeandle (2011) reported that carers do find the role positive in that is provided a sense of family, community and friendship. It is therefore important that the positives of caring for a loved one are not overlooked and the valuable care they provide is recognised, encouraged and actively supported. This may mean a number of different things- from respite, to provision of support networks of their own, to a simple word of acknowledgment and appreciation from professionals.

Conclusion

Health care professionals may overlook psychosocial aspects of an individual with a wound due to the main focus being on the clinical aspects of wound care. However, this oversight may be problematic as social support can improve healing, mental and physical health, acts as a buffer against stressors, and improves patients' well-being. Hence, improving the social support opportunities for those with a wound may prove beneficial not only for the psychological health of the individual patient but also for their physical health. Furthermore, as the number of individuals with chronic wounds may be on the increase community based intervention may be preferable and could contribute to overall management of those with a wound. The promotion of social support will not only enhance psychosocial well-being but may also improve wound healing rate. A number of such models are available and show promise but need to be formally investigated in order to be widely introduced for this reason alone.

In contrast, there is limited research that explores the impact of chronic wounds on the family and, in particular, to the partner of the individual with the wound. This is unfortunate given the key role that family members play in supporting successful adaptation to chronic disorders. Although parallels can be drawn from other conditions this is an area that warrants further investigation. Drawing from other chronic conditions it would appear that there could be significant burden on the spouse or other family members which may bring with it significant physical and psychological morbidity which needs to be addressed in order that not only that their health can be protected but the individual patient can continue to be supported with their own health concerns.

References

Aoun SM, Kristjanson LJ, Currow DC, Hudson PL. Caregiving for the terminally ill: at what cost? Palliat Med. 2005;19:551–5.

Aranda S, Hayman-White L. Home caregivers of the person with advanced cancer: an Australian perspective. Cancer Nurs. 2001;24(4):1–7.

Baanders AN, Heijmans MJWM. The impact of chronic disease. Fam Community Health. 2007;30:305–17.

Baharestani MM. The lived experience of wives caring for their frail, homebound, elderly husbands with pressure ulcers. Adv Wound Care. 1994;7(3):40–2, 44–6, 50 passim.

Bennett JM, Fagundes CP, Kiecolt-Glaser JK. The chronic stress of caregiving accelerates the natural aging of the immune system. In Immunosenescence. New York: Springer; 2013. p. 35-46.

Berkman LF. The Role of Social Relations in Health Promotion. Psychosom Med. 1995;57(3):245–54.

Berkman LF, Syme LS. Social networks, host resistance, and mortality: a nine-year follow-up study of Alameda county residents. Am J Epidemiol. 1979;109(2):186–204.

Brown G. Long-term outcomes of full-thickness pressure ulcers: Healing and mortality. Ostomy Wound Manage. 2003;49(10):42–50.

Brown A. Chronic leg ulcers, part 1: do they affect a patient's social life? Br J Nurs. 2005a;14(17):894–8.

Brown A. Chronic leg ulcers, part 2: do they affect a patient's social life? Br J Nurs. 2005b;14(18):986–9.

Brown G. Speech to the volunteering conference, London, 2005c. 31 Jan 2005.

Brown A. Does social support impact on venous ulcer healing or recurrence? Br J Community Nurs. 2008;13(3 Suppl):S8–15.

Brown A. Managing chronic venous leg ulcers part 2: time for a new pragmatic approach? J Wound Care. 2010;19(3):85–95.

Brummett BH, Barefoot JC, Siegler IC, Clapp-Channing NE, Lytle BL, Bosworth HB, Williams Jr RB, Mark DB. Characteristics of socially isolated patients with coronary artery disease who are

at elevated risk for mortality. Psychosom Med. 2001;63: 267–72.
Buckner L, Yeandle S. Calculating the value of carers' support. Carers UK Report; London: Carers UK; 2011. p. 15. ISBN 978 1 873747 02 5.
Charles H. The Lindsay leg club model. EWMA J. 2010;10(3):38–40.
Cohen S. Psychosocial models of the role of social support in the etiology of physical disease. Health Psychol. 1988;7(3):269.
Cohen L, Manion L, Morrison K. Research Methods in Education. 5th ed. London: Routledge Falmer; 2000.
Coyne JC, Smith DA. Couples coping with a myocardial infarction: A contextual perspective on wives' distress. J Pers Soc Psychol. 1991;61(3):404–12.
Detillion CE, Craft TK, Glasper ER, Prendergast BJ, DeVries AC. Social facilitation of wound healing. Psychoneuroendocrinology. 2004;29(8):1004–11.
Douglas V. Living with a chronic leg ulcer: an insight into patients' experiences and feelings. J Wound Care. 2001;10(9):355–60.
Edwards H, Courtney M, Finlayson K, et al. Improved healing rates for chronic venous leg ulcers: Pilot study results from a randomized controlled trial of a community nursing intervention. Int J Nurs Pract. 2005;11:169–76.
Edwards H, Courtney M, Finlayson K, Shuter P, Lindsay E. A randomised controlled trial of a community nursing intervention: improved quality of life and healing for clients with chronic leg ulcers. J Clin Nurs. 2009;18(11):1541–9.
Ell K. Social networks, social support, and coping with serious illness: The family connection. Soc Sci Med. 1996;42(2):173–83.
Ertel KA, Glymour MM, Berkman LF. Social networks and health: a life course perspective integrating observational and experimental evidence. J Soc Personal Relationships. 2009;26(1):73–92.
Everson-Rose SA, Lewis TT. Psychosocial factors and cardiovascular diseases. Annu Rev Public Health. 2005;26:469–500.
Finlayson K, Edwards H, Courtney M. Relationships between preventive activities, psychosocial factors and recurrence of venous leg ulcers: a prospective study. J Adv Nurs. 2011;67(10):2180–90.
Frasure-Smith N, Lesp'erance F, Gravel G, Masson A, Juneau M, Talajic M, Bourassa MG. Social support, depression, and mortality during the first year after myocardial infarction. Circulation. 2000;101:1919–24.
Freeman E, Gibbins A, Walker M, Hapeshi J. 'Look after your legs': patients' experience of an assessment clinic. Br J Community Nurs. 2007;12(Sup1):S19–25.

Gibbons C, Dempster M, Moutray M. Stress, coping and satisfaction in nursing students. J Adv Nurs. 2011;67(3):621–32.

Glasdam S, Timm H, Vittrup R. Support efforts for caregivers of chronically ill persons. Clin Nurs Res. 2010;19:233–65.

Gleeson-Kreig J, Bernal H, Woolley S. The role of social support in the self-management of diabetes mellitus among a Hispanic population. Public Health Nurs. 2002;19:215–22.

Gordon L, Edwards H, Courtney M, Finlayson K, Shuter P, Lindsay E. A cost-effectiveness analysis of two community models of nursing care for managing chronic venous leg ulcers. J Wound Care. 2006;15(8):348.

Gore S. Stress-buffering functions of social supports: An appraisal and clarification of research models. In: Dohrenwend B, Dohrenwend B, editors. Stressful life events and their context. New York: Prodist; 1981. p. 202–22.

Harker J. Influences on patient adherence with compression hosiery. J Wound Care. 2000;9(8):379–82.

Helgeson VS. Social support and quality of life. Qual Life Res. 2003;12(1):25–31.

Heinen M, Borm G, van der Vleuten C, Evers A, Oostendorp R, van Achterberg T. The Lively Legs self-management programme increased physical activity and reduced wound days in leg ulcer patients: Results from a randomized controlled trial. Int J Nurs Stud. 2012;49:151–61.

Herber OR, Schnepp W, Rieger MA. A systematic review on the impact of leg ulceration on patients' quality of life. Health Qual Life Outcomes. 2007;5(44):1–12.

Hibbard JH, Pope CR. The quality of social roles as predictors of morbidity and mortality. Soc Sci Med. 1993;36:217–25.

Holt-Lunstad J, Smith TB, Layton JB. Social relationships and mortality risk: A meta-analytic review. PLoS Med. 2010;7(7): e1000316.

Hopkins A. Disrupted lives: investigating coping strategies for non-healing leg ulcers. Br J Nurs. 2004a;13(9):556–63.

Hopkins A. The use of qualitative research methodologies to explore leg ulceration. J Tissue Viability. 2004b;14(4):142–7.

Hopkins A, Dealey C, Bale S, DeFloor T, Worboys F. Patient stories of living with a pressure ulcer. J Adv Nurs. 2006;56(4):345–53.

Johansson S, Fahlstršm G. Good intentions. Vardi Norden. 1993;13:15–22.

Jones JE, Robinson J, Barr W, Carlisle C. Impact of exudate and odour from chronic venous leg ulceration. Nurs Stand. 2008a;22(45):53–61.

Jones RA, Taylor AG, Bourguignon C. Family interactions among African American Prostate Cancer Survivors. Fam Community Health. 2008b;31(3):213–20.

Keeling D, et al. Social support some pragmatic implications for health care professionals. J Adv Nurs. 1996;23(1):76–81.

Kiecolt-Glaser JK, Newton TL. Marriage and health: his and hers. Psychol Bull. 2001;127:472–503.

Kiecolt-Glaser JK, Marucha PT, Malarkey WB, Mercado AM, Glaser R. Slowing of wound healing by psychological stress. Lancet. 1995;346:1194–6.

Kiecolt-Glaser JK, McGuire L, Robles TF, Glaser R. Psychoneuroimmunology: psychological influences on immune function and health. J Consult Clin Psychol. 2002;70:537–47.

Lee M, Rotheram-Borus MJ. Challenges associated with increased survival among parents living with HIV. Am J Public Health. 2001;91:1303–9.

Lewis MA, Rook KS. Social control in personal relationships: Impact on health behaviors and psychological distress. Health Psychol. 1999;18:63–71.

Li R, Cooper C, Bradley J, Shulman A, Livingston G. Coping strategies and psychological morbidity in family carers of people with dementia: a systematic review and meta-analysis. J Affect Disord. 2011;139:1–11.

Lin N. Conceptualizing social support. In: Lin N, Dean A, Ensel W, editors. Social support, life events, and depression. New York: Academic; 1986. p. 17–30.

Lindsay E. Leg clubs: A new approach to patient-centred leg ulcer management. Nurs Health Sci. 2000;2(3):139–41.

Lindsay E. The Lindsay Leg Club a model for evidence-based leg ulcer management. Br J Community Nurs. 2004;9(6 Suppl):S15–20.

Lindsay E. Legging it to the Club. Pract Manage. 2008;18(3):26–7.

Lindsay E. Changing policy and practice to empower older people living with chronic wounds. Symposium abstract; The 20th IAGG World congress of gerontology and geriatrics, Korea. 2013.

Maida V, et al. Symptoms associated with malignant wounds: a prospective case series. J Pain Symptom Manage. 2009;37(2):206–11.

Manne SL, Zautra AJ. Couples coping with chronic illness. J Behav Med. 1990;13:327–42.

McDonald J, Hayes L. Promoting resilience in young people: progress in implementing a framework in schools. Health Promot J Austr. 2001;12:261–4.

Moffatt CJ, Franks PJ, Doherty DC, et al. Socio-demographic factors in chronic leg ulceration. Br J Dermatol. 2006;155(2):307–12.

Moffatt C, Kommala D, Dourdin N, Choe Y. Venous leg ulcers: patient concordance with compression therapy and its impact on healing and prevention of recurrence. Int Wound J. 2009;6:386–93.

Moos RH, Moos BS. Manual for Familiy Environment Scale. Palo Alto: Consulting Psychologists Press; 1981.

Munro I, Edward KL. The burden of care of gay male carers caring for men living with HIV/AIDS. Am J Mens Health. 2010;4:287.

Oddone CG, Hybels CF, McQuid DR, Steffens DC. Social support modifies the relationship between personality and depressive symptoms in older adults. Am J Geriatr Psychiatry. 2011;19(2):123–31.

Oehlenslaeger B. You miss the one you still got. Special Poedagogik. 1998;18:104–13.

Ousey KJ, Gillibrand W, Stephenson J. Achieving international consensus for the prevention of orthopaedic wound blistering: results of a Delphi survey. Int Wound J. 2013;10(2):177–84.

Ozbay F, Johnson DC, Dimoulas E, Morgan III CA, Charney D, Southwick S. Social support and resilience to stress: from neurobiology to clinical practice. Psychiatry (Edgmont). 2007;4(5):35.

Parker PD, Lüdtke O, Trautwein U, Roberts B. Personality and relationship quality during the transition from high school to early adulthood. J Pers. 2012;80:1061–81.

Persoon A, Heinen M, van der Vleuten C, de Rooij M, van de Kerkhof P, van Achterberg T. Leg ulcers: a review of their impact on daily life. J Clin Nurs. 2004;13(3):341–54.

Price P, et al. Why combine a foam dressing with ibuprofen for wound pain and moist wound healing? Int Wound J. 2007;4(S1):1–3.

Quick JD, Nelson DL, Matuszek PA, Whittington JL, Quick JC. Social support, secure attachments, and health. In: Cooper CL, editor. Handbook of stress, medicine, and health. Boca Raton: CRC Press; 1996. p. 269–87.

Rees J, O'Boyle CA, MacDonagh R. Quality of life. J R Soc Med. 2001;94:563–6.

Riemsma RP, Taal E, et al. The burden of care for informal caregivers of patients with rheumatoid arthritis. Psychol Health. 1999;14:773–94.

Russell D, Cutrona CE, Rose J, Yurko K. Social and emotional loneliness: an examination of Weiss's typology of loneliness. J Pers Soc Psychol. 1984;46(6):1313.

Sales E. Family burden and quality of life. Qual Life Res. 2003;12(1):33–41.

Sapolsky R. Why Zebras Don't Get Ulcers: A Guide to Stress, Stress-Related Diseases and Coping. 3rd ed. New York: Holt; 2004.

Sarason BR. Social support, social behaviour and cognitive processes. In: Schwartzer R, editor. Self regulated cognitions in anxiety and motivation. Hillsdale: Lawrence Erlbaum; 1986. p. 71–86.

Sarason IG, Levine HM, Basham RB, Sarason BR. Assessing social support: The social support questionnaire. J Pers Soc Psychol. 1983;44:127–39.

Sarason IG, Sarason BR, Shearin EN, Pierce GR. A brief measure of social support: Practical and theoretical implications. J Soc Pers Relationships. 1987;4(4):497–510.

Sherbourne CD, Stewart AL. The MOS social support survey. Soc Sci Med. 1991;32(6):705–14.

Shuter P, Finlayson K, Edwards H, Courtney MH, Herbert C, Lindsay E. Leg Clubs – Beyond the ulcers: case studies based on participatory action research. Wound Pract Res. 2011;19(1):16–20.

Solowiej K, Upton D. Take it easy: how the cycle of stress and pain associated with wound care affects recovery. Nurs Residential Care. 2010a;12(9):443–6.

Solowiej K, Upton D. The assessment and management of pain and stress in wound care. Br J Community Nurs. 2010b;15(6):S26–33.

Soubhi H, Fortin M, Hudson C. Perceived conflict in the couple and chronic illness management. BMC Fam Practit. 2006;7:59.

Spence A, Hasson F, Waldron M, et al. Active carers: living with chronic obstructive pulmonary disease. Int J Palliat Nurs. 2008;14(8):368–72.

Thoits PA. Stress and Health: Major Findings and Policy Implications. J Health Soc Behav. 2010;51:S41.

Thoits PA. Mechanisms linking social ties and support to physical and mental health. J Health Soc Behav. 2011;52(2):145–61.

Thomas C, Morris SM, Harman JC. Companions through cancer: the care given by informal carers in cancer contexts. Soc Sci Med. 2002;54:529–44.

Toshima MT, Kaplan RM, Ries AL. Experimental evaluation of rehabilitation in chronic obstructive pulmonary disease: short-term effects on exercise endurance and health status. Health Psychol. 1990;9(3):237.

Trief PM, Sandberg J, Greenberg RP, et al. Describing support: a qualitative study of couples living with diabetes. Fam Syst Health. 2003;21(1):57–67.

Troup CL, Dewe PL. Exploring the nature of control and its role in the appraisal of workplace stress. Work Stress. 2002;16:335–55.

Uchino BN. Social support and physical health: Understanding the health consequences of relationships. New Haven: Yale University Press; 2004.

Uchino BN. Social support and health: a review of physiological processes potentially underlying links to disease outcomes. J Behav Med. 2006;29(4):377–87.

Umberson D. Family status and health behaviors: Social control as a dimension of social integration. J Health Soc Behav. 1987;28(3):306–19.

Umberson D, Montez JK. Social relationships and health: a flashpoint for health policy. J Health Soc Behav. 2010;51:S54–66.

Upton D, Andrews A. Negative Pressure Wound Therapy: Improving the Patient Experience, Part Two of Three. J Wound Care. 2013a;22(11):582–91.

Upton D, Andrews A. Negative Pressure Wound Therapy: Improving the Patient Experience, Part One of Three. J Wound Care. 2013b;22(10):552–7.

Upton D, Andrews A. Pain and trauma in negative pressure wound therapy: a review. Int Wound J. 2013c; Advance online publication.

Vermeiden J, Doorn L, Da Costa AMD, Kaptein AA, Steenvoorde P. Coping strategies used by patients with chronic and/or complex wounds. Wounds. 2009;21(12):324–8.

Victor CR, Scambler S, Shah S, Cook DG, Harris T, Rink E, de Wilde S. Has loneliness amongst older people increased? An investigation into variations between cohorts. Ageing Soc. 2002;22(1):1–13.

Vitaliano PP, et al. Is caregiving hazardous to one's physical health? A meta-analysis. Psychol Bull. 2003;129(6):946–72.

Weller CD, Buchbinder R, Johnston RV. Interventions for helping people adhere to compression treatments for venous leg ulceration. Cochrane Database Syst Rev. 2013;(9):CD008378.

White Y, Greyner B. The bio-psychosocial impact of end-stage renal disease: The experience of dialysis patients and their partners. J Adv Nurs. 1999;30(6):1312–20.

Wise G. The social ulcer. Nurs Times. 1986;82(21):47–9.

Wissing U, Ek AC, Unosson M. A follow-up study of ulcer healing, nutrition, and life-situation in elderly patients with leg ulcers. J Nutr Health Aging. 2001;5(1):37–42.

Woods B. Promoting well-being and independence for people with dementia. Int J Geriatr Psychiatry. 1999;14:97–109.

Zimet GD, Dahlem NW, Zimet SG, Farley GK. The Multidimensional Scale of Perceived Social Support. J Pers Assess. 1988;52:30–41.

Chapter 9
Conclusion

> Box 9.1: Key Points
> - The economic costs of wound care can be extensive and account for a significant proportion of health service costs;
> - Despite the significant financial costs, the psychological consequences can be just as important and costly;
> - Pain, stress, mood disorders, well-being, concordance, social support are all fundamental psychological issues that the practicing clinician should consider to develop their wound care practice;
> - Patient well-being should be at the centre of all clinical practice;
> - It is imperative that the clinician incorporates psychological knowledge and skills into their everyday practice for the benefit of all their patients.

Summary

Psychological stress, pain, negative emotions, malodour, high exudate levels, social isolation, sleep and mobility problems are just some of the negative consequences of living with a wound. The subsequent psychological effects can have a severe impact on an individual's quality of life and their well-being. The evidence suggests that these psychological factors not only influence the occurrence of further wounds, but they also exacerbate the severity of a wound and affect its ability to heal, resulting in the individual having to endure further psychological problems as a consequence- a vicious circle that clinicians must be aware of when treating patients with wounds. This chapter explores some of the negative consequences of a wound and how some psychological resources can help both the clinician and, more importantly, the patient and their family. Summarizing the material presented elsewhere in this book and highlighting the clinical relevance, this chapter demonstrates the importance of psychology in both the experience of living with a wound and effective wound care.

Introduction

Chronic wounds have been described as: "*a silent epidemic that affects a large fraction of the world population and poses a major and gathering threat to the public health and economy*" (Sen et al. 2009, p. 763). It has been estimated that there are over 200,000 patients with chronic wounds in the UK (Posnett and Franks 2007) although this figure, despite being frequently cited, is probably a significant under-estimate. With an aging population and increasing incidence of concomitant factors, such as obesity and diabetes, it is possible that this figure has increased considerably since their report and will continue to do so.

The cost in the UK to the NHS of these chronic wounds has been estimated at £2–3 billion: approximately 3 % of NHS budget (Posnett and Franks 2007). The health care costs of chronic wounds in the European population accounted for 2 % of the European health budget (Bottrich 2014). In the Scandinavian countries, the costs of chronic wounds comprised 2–4 % of the total health care expenditure (Gottrup et al. 2001). Graves and Zheng (2014) suggest that in Australia the direct health care costs reach approximately US$2.85 billion.

Whatever country, continent or service, wounds are a significant cost to the respective health economies. The elements included in these estimates tend to focus on the medical costs alone. Hence, these have been included: costs of dressing materials, average hospitalisation rates, average time to healing, and complication rates have all been considered. However, an aspect that is often overlooked is the cost of the psychological consequences of the wounds: both to the patient and the health service (see Box 9.1). The psychological consequences of living with a chronic wound can include many negative emotions, such as stress, anxiety, concern about physical symptoms, lack of self-worth and feelings of despair. These can vary in severity, from minor negative emotions to suicidal thoughts, depending on each individual case (Upton and South 2011; Upton et al. 2012a, b, c). Upton and Hender (2012) explored the economic costs of the additional psychosocial problems with wound care and suggested that in the UK these additional cost of treating chronic wound patients for mood disorder could be as much as £85.5 million per annum as a lower estimate.

At the outset of this book we highlighted the growing research interest in psychological issues in health care and wound care in particular. It would appear that this interest can have a financial reality as well. For many years, health care professionals may have overlooked some of the important psychosocial aspects of an individual's care but this situation is changing and we hope that this book has gone someway to strengthening the time and energy afforded these variables. In this way not only the economic factors can be addressed but also, more importantly, the needs of the patient.

When constantly dealing with many wound patients in a time and resourced pressed environment, it may be difficult for practitioners to fully appreciate the impact a chronic wound can have upon an individuals' life. The focus can often be directed towards treating the wound rather than the associated sequelea (Briggs and Flemming 2007). We hope that this book has highlighted how some of the research evidence may be of particular relevance to the health care professional in their day-to-day practice.

Studies have also shown that patients living with long-term wounds often have poor psychological wellbeing and a reduced quality of life as a consequence of the impact of the wound and wound care. The impact on the patient and their caregiver's social life can be extensive and all encompassing.

The presence of these factors, along with immobility, social isolation, pain, mood disorders and other psychosocial factors not only exacerbates their severity and jeopardises their ability to heal but also could lead to further wounds occurrence. Of course, there are some protective factors and these can include not only positive and appropriate clinical wound care but also psychosocial factors.

Each of these factors, whether positive or negative, has been described, evidenced and reported in this book. This final chapter will emphasise the clinical relevance of the material presented and provide some simple implications for professional practice (see Table 9.1).

TABLE 9.1 Psychological factors and relevance to care

Factor	Element	Some implications for the clinician
Psychosocial	Lack of energy	Education
	Work limitations	Support
	Leisure activity restrictions	Cognitive therapy
	Low self-esteem	Acknowledgement of difficulties
	Daily routine alterations	Development of coping strategies
	Sleep disturbance	Social support development
	Body image distortion	
	Fatigue	
	Restricted mobility,	
	Odour and social isolation	
	Depression	
	Anxiety	
	Mood disorders	

Table 9.1 (continued)

Factor	Element	Some implications for the clinician
Pain	Pain from wound	Cognitive behaviour therapy
	Pain from treatment	Distraction techniques
	Background pain	Imagery
	Pain from anticipation of treatment	Relaxation
		Altering significance of the pain
		P.A.I.N model
		Appropriate clinical techniques
		Acknowledgement of pain
Stress	Stress from pain	Pain management techniques
	Stress from treatment	Calm and relaxed treatment environment
	Stress from psychosocial issues	Cognitive behaviour therapy
	Stress delayed healing	Education and appropriate control
		Self-management
		Appropriate dressings
		Pre-information for novel treatments

Psychosocial Issues of Wounds

As we have seen in Chap. 1, most researchers, clinicians and patients agree there are a host of psychosocial factors that can affect the individual patient of which the health care professional should be aware. These can include: lack of energy, limitations in work and leisure activities, worries and frustrations, a lack of self-esteem, frequency and regularity of dressing changes, which affect a patient's daily routine, feeling of continued fatigue due to lack of adequate sleep, restricted mobility, persistent pain, exudate, odour and social isolation (Upton and South 2011). Mobility restrictions may effect every aspect of the patients life, limiting their availability to work or perform household tasks. Even attending to personal hygiene may become difficult, as previously independent patients become reliant on others and report loss of self-worth and role reversal within families. Social isolation may be exacerbated by the impact on self-esteem of the physical consequences of the wound- the odour, any strike-through or required dressing changes. These may increase anxiety and depression, embarrassment, negative body image and social isolation, which can all impact negatively on quality of life (Hareendran et al. 2005; Herber et al. 2007).

All of these factors may contribute to the psychological distress experienced by both the patient and their carer. Furthermore, some individuals may try different methods of coping with the physical manifestation of the wound. Such actions are often ineffective and, in some cases, can worsen the condition of the wound. For example, Lo et al. (2008) reported the experiences of cancer patients living with a malignant fungating wound. Findings suggest that some patients would attempt to cover wounds to avoid leakage, would drink less fluid in the hope of reducing the amount of exudate produced and would remove bandages to help exudate disperse. Patients often feel embarrassed about exudate leakage and malodour and have difficulty maintaining dignity and outward appearances (Walshe 1995; Hyde et al. 1999).

It is therefore essential that the clinician recognises and responds to these psychosocial issues: dealing with any self-esteem issues, any psychological distress or social isolation and importantly providing accurate information and education for the patient to reduce any misunderstanding or inappropriate coping mechanisms. In this way it should be possible to promote a positive approach to the patient's situation and their treatment. This may involve information on self-management, self-care, and social integration (see Table 9.1).

Pain

In a systematic review of studies on the impact of leg ulcers on daily life Persoon et al. (2004) listed pain as the first and most dominant factor and this has been fully explored in Chap. 2. Jones et al. (2006) found prolonged pain (along with malodour) was the specific symptom associated with anxiety and depression. Given the numerous negative effects of pain, it is not surprising that healthcare practitioners unanimously believed that reducing chronic wound pain could improve patients' psychological state significantly (Upton et al. 2012a, b, c). However, in an interactive wound care survey of 246 wound conference delegates only 35 % of NHS community staff and 44 % of NHS hospital staff considered that wound pain was being addressed sufficiently (Lloyd Jones et al. 2010). Given the over-riding significance of pain, the reported poor support provided and the potential impact that pain may have on treatment concordance, stress levels and ultimately wound healing it is the key issue that clinicians have to address in wound care through careful assessment and management. Along with the underlying wound aetiologies and local trauma that is exacerbated at dressing change (Woo and Sibbald 2008), a constellation of patient factors including emotions, personality structure and stress are integral to the comprehensive assessment and management of wound related pain. These can all be encapsulated under the P.A.I.N. (Preparation, Assessment, Intervention and Normalisation) model previously described (see Chap. 2).

There are many psychological therapies that can help the patient deal with their pain. For example, cognitive therapy that aims to modify attitudes, beliefs, and expectations has been shown to be successful in the management of both stress and pain. Furthermore, distraction techniques, imagery, relaxation or altering the significance of the pain to an individual can also be successful in reducing pain. Patients can also learn relaxation exercises to help reduce anxiety related tension in the muscle that contributes to pain. These techniques can be employed by the clinician, or referred on for more specialist interventions and can help not only pain but stress and other psychological disorders. Finally, support from others, whether those with a similar condition or from the family can help and should be actively encouraged by the clinician (see Table 9.1).

Stress

A systematic review and meta-analysis (Walburn et al. 2009) explored the relationship between stress on a variety of wound types in different contexts (for example, different types of acute and chronic wounds and experimentally created wounds such as punch biopsies). The findings demonstrated that the relationship between stress and wound healing is clinically relevant (Kiecolt-Glaser et al. 1995; Cole-King and Harding 2001). For example, in a study of 72 patients with burns, it was found that the greater the level of distress a person was under, the slower the wound healing process can be (Wilson et al. 2011). This study, along with many others and other clinically relevant reviews (e.g. Solowiej et al. 2010a, b; Solowiej et al. 2010; Solowiej and Upton 2010a, b; Upton and Solowiej 2011) presented in detail in Chap. 3 demonstrates the importance of minimising the stress of both living with a wound and the wound management regime.

Wound-related pain at dressing changes has also been shown to correlate positively with stress and anxiety (Solowiej et al. 2009, 2010a, b). The relationship between pain and anxiety could be due to the patient being more sensitive to pain due to increased anxiety and fear, particularly if this is based on a past experience (Mudge et al. 2008; Woo 2010). Alternatively, patients suffering higher pain levels are more likely to become stressed and anxious. This may, in turn, impact on their healing rate. Considerable evidence now exists demonstrating the link between stress and delayed healing and controlling pain more effectively can affect stress and should also impact upon healing rates (Cole-King and Harding 2001; Soon and Acton 2006; Woo 2010; Gouin and Kiecolt-Glaser 2011; Solowiej and Upton 2010a, b). Consequently this has considerable implications for practice. It may be that the continued stress of wound care change leads to chronic stress. In this way, stress has a cumulative

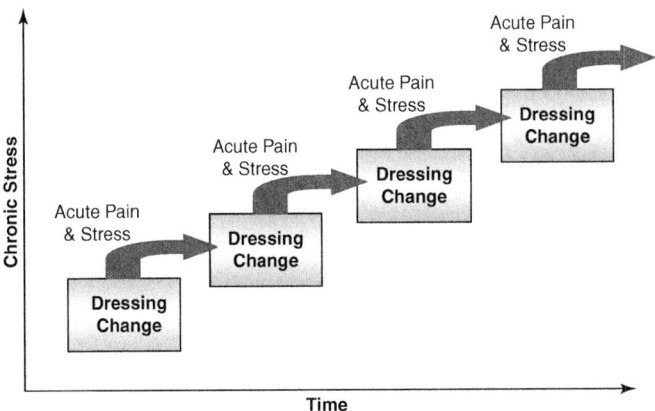

FIGURE 9.1 A potential relationship between acute pain and stress occurring at dressing change and increased chronic stress levels

impact- the "minor hassle" or relatively low levels of pain experienced at any one dressing change have a significant impact over time (see Fig. 9.1).

Practitioners have to appreciate this cumulative impact and minimise stress and pain at all wound changes. This may be related to dressing choice, relaxed and calm environments, effective communication with the patient, provision of appropriate support, or demonstrated psychological or physical therapies (see Table 9.1).

Quality of Life and Well-Being

Although there have been a wealth of studies exploring the quality of life (QoL) of patients with wounds, many tend to focus on 'health-related quality of life' (HRQoL) or 'health status'. Such measures are useful as outcome measures of treatment, yet they do not always tell us about important psychological factors and the impact of wounds on well-being; consequently, these issues are often overlooked (Upton et al. 2013a, b). Throughout this book we have attempted to address these psychological factors and put well-being at the centre of the discussions (see Fig. 9.2).

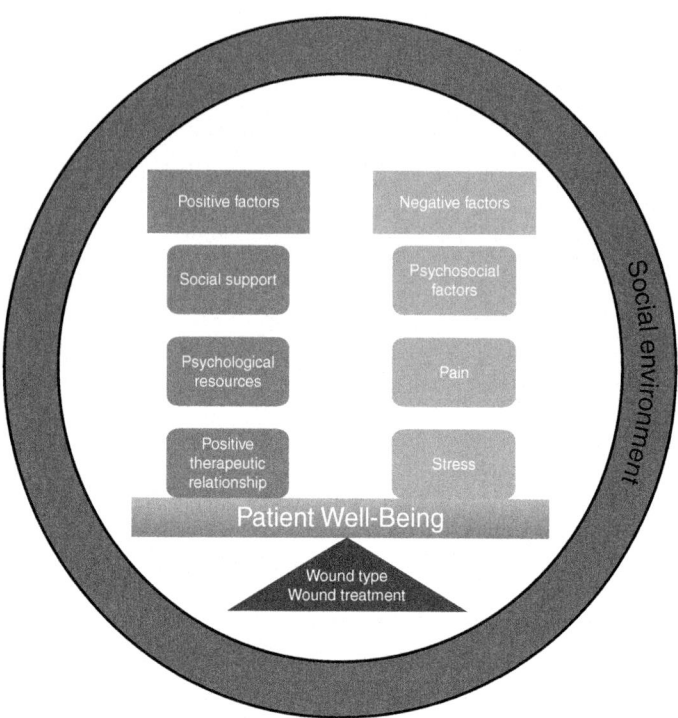

Figure 9.2 Central importance of patient well-being

The well-being of patients is a fundamental issue to be considered in wound care, with a holistic approach to treatment needed (Maddox 2012). Research has shown that many healthcare professionals are often aware of the complex issues that patients experience, yet they cannot always address these due to time constraints and a focus on achieving clinical outcomes (e.g. Hollinworth and Hawkins 2002). Furthermore, clinicians and patients may have different priorities during treatment, with clinical staff working towards healing, whilst the primary concern of patients is often relief from symptoms such as pain, discomfort and psychosocial difficulties (Husband 2001; Brown 2005a, b, c; Maddox 2012).

The patient-health care professional relationship is often very positive for people with wounds, and these interactions may protect and promote their well-being. However, interactions that are perceived to be negative may have the opposite effect, and clinicians may not always able to address psychosocial issues with patients due to the focus on treatment and healing. Consequently, important issues may not receive the attention they need, leading to poorer well-being and potentially lower treatment concordance and a prolonged healing process. It is hoped that this book has emphasised the importance of these psychological variables in the treatment of the patient with a wound. This is irrespective of wound or treatment type, since the chapters have demonstrated that psychological variables can play an important role in either promoting or delaying wound healing. In this way, the focus on psychological well-being should not be viewed as incompatible with improved clinical outcomes. Indeed, it can be seen as complementary- improving well-being not only improves psychological outcomes but also the patient's clinical outcome (see Chap. 4).

Different Wound and Psychological Outcomes

Chapter 5 explored different wound types and how psychological variables may be related to each of these. Burns, Diabetic Foot Ulcers, Venous Leg Ulcers and Pressure Ulcers were also explored, and key factors and condition specific variables detailed. It was evident that although there were many similarities in some psychological factors associated with the wounds there were also significant differences. For example, in burn injuries it is important to recognise that there may be some pre-existing psychological morbidity. Obviously the clinician must recognise that this is at a population level rather than an individual level. That is, the group of patients with burns have higher levels of pre-existing psychological morbidity compared to other groups. At a patient level, all should be treated individually with appropriate assessment and intervention.

Of course with most chronic conditions, prevention is better than cure. It is better to prevent pressure ulcers than to deal with them, it is better to prevent DFU rather than deal with the psychological and physical consequences, it is better to prevent burns rather than deal with them. A fundamental issue underlying any prevention message is one of education (Upton and Thirlaway 2013). For example, for people at risk from DFU education is recommended, combined with other preventive measures (International Working Group on the Diabetic Foot 2007). However, some evidence suggests that a group based educational session may not be successful for re-ulceration prevention although there is some evidence that it can prevent ulcers developing in the first place (Annersten Gershater et al. 2011). Again, prevention is better than cure. It may be that it requires more than simple education messages and that a multi-modal psycho-educational programme may have more of an impact (e.g. Vedhara et al. 2012).

Furthermore, it is not just the patient that may benefit from education. Educating health care professionals involved in the patient's daily life and also educating the patient's next of kin may constitute a more effective intervention and this can be applied across many wound types. Hence, if compression bandages were applied consistently and correctly then concordance might improve as would wound healing. If family members and spouses were educated then the negative psychological consequences of treatment might be reduced and concordance improved. Hence, psycho-education (such as that described in Chap. 5) might prove beneficial in recovery by improving both the concordance to the different treatment types available and reducing any psychological distress associated with the condition and treatment.

Different Treatments and Psychological Outcomes

Irrespective of the form of treatment, Fletcher (2008) presents a 'best practice statement care pathway' suggesting wounds should be cared for in a standardised way, with clear objectives, regular reviews and onward referral to specialist when patients are not progressing as expected. She advocates wound care should address every need of the patient in order to maximise their quality of life, taking an holistic approach which may involve addressing concurrent issues such as under-nutrition, illness and infection and their social environment. Listening to, and involving patients in a collaborative care plan with appropriate goals is also important (Dowsett 2008) and may help reduce the incidence of psychological distress and improve physical health (see Table 9.2). Understanding the needs of the patient, utilising the most appropriate treatment regime to achieve improved healing are vitally important to help patients cope and avoid the devastating effects that can delay healing.

Health care professionals need to ensure that any treatment regime follows best practice guidance and that any

TABLE 9.2 Protective factors for dealing with the psychosocial issues associated with wounds

Factor	Element	Some implications for the clinician
Social support	Reducing stress	Development of social support mechanisms
	Improving adaptation	Dealing with any carer issues
	Improving concordance	
	Carer burden	
Communication	Positive therapeutic relationship	Psycho-educational programmes
	Education and self-care	Understanding of social context
		Knowledge and understanding
Concordance	Knowledge, satisfaction and recall	Self-care
		Education
		Positive clinician-patient relationship

potential psychological consequences are recognised and dealt with appropriately. Similarly, some treatments may reduce psychological distress whereas others may increase it- clinicians have to assess individual patients and their interaction with their treatments to ensure negative consequences are minimized. For example, although many of the techniques and treatments may be familiar to the clinician they may not be common to the patient that may result in increased pain and anxiety experienced by the patient, which needs to be addressed. This may be of particular concern with novel treatments such as NPWT as presented in Chap. 6.

In order for any treatment to be effective, of course, it is essential that the patient follow the advice of the clinician. Enhancing concordance through a positive therapeutic relationship is essential in order for effective treatments that, in itself, can promote healing. This may involve a number of positive practices: using the correct technique, communicating effectively, providing education and information, reducing anxiety and having a positive therapeutic technique.

Communication and Concordance

A positive therapeutic relationship between the health practitioner and the patient can enhance treatment concordance, which can, itself, improve patient outcomes (Ebbeskog and Emami 2005; Morgan et al. 2004). As a first step to cultivating a positive relationship, clinicians need to clearly acknowledge that both stress and pain are frequently experienced at dressing changes. Clear information to patients that these symptoms are part of a normal response is essential, although a clinical goal should be to minimize the experience of these symptoms. Education is a key strategy to empower patients and to improve wound related pain control. Only a small proportion of patients are aware of factors contributing to their chronic wounds and treatment strategies to improve their conditions (Chase et al. 1997). In a pilot study (Gibson et al. 2004), five chronic wound patients described dressing change pain more manageable after receiving educational information. Pain related education is a necessary step in effecting change in pain management by rebuking common misconceptions and myth that may obstruct effective pain management.

The patient-professional relationship has been discussed in a number of studies, with most demonstrating the positive effect that this contact has on well-being. For example, the patients in Hopkins' (2004a, b) study reported feeling happy and able to joke with nurses once relationships had formed. They felt understood and enjoyed these interactions. However, this was not the case when unfamiliar nurses provided their care. Similar findings have emerged from other studies (e.g. Byrne and Kelly 2010; Walshe 1995; Brown 2005a, b, c). The central importance of the clinician-patient relationship cannot be under-estimated in the successful treatment of both clinical and psychological variables. It is therefore essential that time, energy and resources are put into developing this. However, the importance of other social support relationships particularly with the family should not be overlooked.

Family and Social Support

Social isolation can also affect social interaction, which may lead to a tendency for patients to keep problems to themselves (Mudge et al. 2008) and this may subsequently increase the stresses and strains of living with a wound with the concomitant impact on healing speed. It has been suggested that social support and emotional disclosure can help the healing process (Klyscz et al. 1998; Gonçalves et al. 2004). For instance, Weinman et al. (2008) found that participants who took part in the emotional disclosure intervention had smaller wounds than control participants at 14 and 21 days. These results suggest that reduced levels of social interaction result in higher levels of perceived stress, which consequently leads patients to have a slower wound-healing time, further affecting their quality of life. Consequently, it is incumbent on the health care professional to ensure that social support is maximized. This may be through a number of means- whether it be the encouragement of family and friend interaction or through attendance at specific social clubs.

For example, attendance at a Leg Club appears to be beneficial for patients and it gives them the opportunity to share their experiences with others who also have ulcers. The importance of patient stories and ensuring that patients are heard has been highlighted by Hawkins and Lindsay (2006). The authors presented a number of patient stories, which tell us how Leg Clubs have empowered patients through educating them about their ulcers and treatment, and making them aware that other people have them too. The patients reported feeling more confident through seeing others make progress and therefore feeling that they could too. These patient stories demonstrate the importance of patient education about their condition and enabling patients to take control and have input into their treatment. The authors also emphasise how patients need to be able to talk about their experiences, and that these need to be learned from and treated as evidence in their own right. In this way, the emotional disclosure suggested by the Weinman et al. (2008) study can occur and, hopefully, healing encouraged.

However, Chap. 8 also explored the negative consequences of living with a wound for the family and, particularly the spouse, of the patient. Carers are a considerable resource to the health economy and to the individual with the wound. It is imperative that the health care professional recognises this value and harnesses it to best effect. This can involve either support for the family, including emotional and practical coping skills, and also education and wound management skills. As such the individual can become an ally in the support of the patient with the wound and thereby improve not only the psychological well-being but also the clinical outcomes.

Conclusion

The painful downward spiral of a wound, negative social consequences, poor well-being and subsequent delayed healing has at its root psychological factors. Similarly, psychological factors can be supportive, protective and enhance wound healing. The centrality of all these factors cannot be underestimated but until recently has tended to be overlooked with the focus being solely on clinical outcomes. It is gratifying that there is now considerable research evidence available that can have a direct and significant impact on patient well-being and wound healing. This book has attempted to highlight and demonstrate the importance of these psychological variables to the individual with the wound and for the clinician in their wound care practice. It is imperative that the practicing clinician takes these factors into account and uses them effectively in their evidence based practice for the benefit of all their patients.

References

Annersten Gershater M, Pilhammar E, Alm Roijer C. Documentation of diabetes care in home nursing service in a Swedish municipality: a cross-sectional study on nurses' documentation. Scand J Caring Sci. 2011;25(2):220–6.

Bottrich JG. Challenges in chronic wound care: the need for interdisciplinary collaboration. 2014. Accessed at: http://medtechviews.eu/article/challenges-chronic-wound-care-need-interdisciplinary-collaboration, on 7 Oct 2014.

Briggs M, Flemming K. Living with leg ulceration: a synthesis of qualitative research. J Adv Nurs. 2007;59(4):319–28.

Brown A. Chronic leg ulcers, part 1: do they affect a patient's social life? Br J Nurs. 2005a;14(17):894–8.

Brown A. Chronic leg ulcers, part 2: do they affect a patient's social life? Br J Nurs. 2005b;14(18):986–9.

Brown G. Speech to the volunteering conference, London, 2005c. 31 Jan 2005.

Byrne O, Kelly M. Living with a chronic leg ulcer. J Community Nurs. 2010;24(5):46–54.

Chase S, Melloni M, Savage A. A forever healing: the lived experience of venous ulcer disease. J Vasc Nurs. 1997;15:73–8.

Cole-King A, Harding KG. Psychological factors and delayed healing in chronic wounds. Psychosom Med. 2001;63:216–20.

Dowsett C. Exudate management: a patient centred approach. J Wound Care. 2008;17(6):249–52.

Ebbeskog B, Emami A. Older patients' experience of dressing changes on venous leg ulcers: more than just a docile patient. J Clin Nurs. 2005;14(10):1223–31.

Fletcher J. Optimising wound care in the UK and Ireland: a best practice statement. Wounds UK. 2008;4(4):73–81.

Gibson MC, Keast D, Woodbury MG, et al. Education intervention in the management of acute procedure-related wound pain: a pilot study. J Wound Care. 2004;13(5):187–90.

Gonçalves ML, de Gouveia Santos VLC, de Mattos Pimenta CA, Suzuki É, Komegae KM. Pain in chronic leg ulcers. J Wound Ostomy Continence Nurs. 2004;31(5):275–83.

Gouin JP, Kiecolt-Glaser JK. The impact of psychological stress on wound healing: methods and mechanisms. Immunol Allergy Clin North Am. 2011;31(1):81–93.

Gottrup F, et al. A new concept of a multidisciplinary wound healing center and a national expert function of wound healing. Arch Surg. 2001;136(7):765–72.

Graves H, Zheng N. Modelling the direct health care costs of chronic wounds in Australia. Wound Prac Res. 2014;22(1):20–33.

Hareendran A, Bradbury A, Budd J, Geroulakos G, Hobbs R, Kenkre J, Symonds T. Measuring the impact of venous leg ulcers on quality of life. J Wound Care. 2005;14(2):53–7.

Hawkins J, Lindsay E. We listen but do we hear? The importance of patient stories. Wound Care. 2006;11(9):S6–14.

Herber OR, Schnepp W, Rieger MA. A systematic review on the impact of leg ulceration on patients' quality of life. Health Qual Life Outcomes. 2007;5(44):1–12.

Hollinworth H, Hawkins J. Teaching nurses psychological support of patients with wounds. Br J Nurs. 2002;11(4 Suppl):S8–18.

Hopkins A. Disrupted lives: investigating coping strategies for non-healing leg ulcers. Br J Nurs. 2004a;13(9):556–63.

Hopkins A. The use of qualitative research methodologies to explore leg ulceration. J Tissue Viability. 2004b;14(4):142–7.

Husband LL. Venous ulceration: the pattern of pain and the paradox. Clin Effectiveness Nurs. 2001;5(1):35–40.

Hyde C, Ward B, Horsfall J, Winder G. Older women's experience of living with chronic leg ulceration. Int J Nurs Pract. 1999;5:189–98.

International Working Group on the Diabetic Foot, Consultative Section of International Diabetes Federation. International Consensus on the Diabetic Foot. Amsterdam: International Working Group on the Diabetic Foot; 2007.

Jones J, Barr W, Robinson J, Carlisle C. Depression in patients with chronic venous ulceration. Br J Nurs. 2006;15(11):17–23.

Kiecolt-Glaser JK, Marucha PT, Malarkey WB, Mercado AM, Glaser R. Slowing of wound healing by psychological stress. Lancet. 1995;346:1194–6.

Klyscz T, Jünger M, Schanz S, Janz M, Rassner G, Kohnen R. Lebensqualität bei chronisch venöser Insuffizienz (CVI). Hautarzt. 1998;49:372–81.

Lloyd Jones M, Greenwood M, Bielby A. Living with wound-associated pain: impact on the patient and what clinicians really think. J Wound Care. 2010;19(8):340–5.

Lo SF, Hu WY, Hayter M, Chang SC, Hsu MY, Wu LY. Experiences of living with a malignant fungating wound: a qualitative study. J Clin Nurs. 2008;17(20):2699–708.

Maddox D. Effects of venous leg ulceration on patients' quality of life. Nurs Stand. 2012;26(38):42–9.

Morgan DA. Formulary of wound management products: a guide for healthcare staff. 9th ed. Surrey: Euromed Communications Ltd; 2004.

Mudge E, Spanou C, Price P. A focus group study into patients' perceptions of chronic wound pain. Wounds UK. 2008;4(2):21–8.

Persoon A, Heinen M, van der Vleuten C, de Rooij M, van de Kerkhof P, van Achterberg T. Leg ulcers: a review of their impact on daily life. J Clin Nurs. 2004;13(3):341–54.

Posnett J, Franks PJ. The costs of skin breakdown and ulceration in the UK. In: Pownall M, editor. Skin breakdown: the silent epidemic. Hull: Smith & Nephew; 2007. p. 6–12.

Sen CK, Gordillo GM, Roy S, Kirsner R, Lambert L, Hunt TK, Longaker MT. Human skin wounds: a major and snowballing threat to public health and the economy. Wound Repair Regen. 2009;17(6):763–71.

Solowiej K, Upton D. Take it easy: how the cycle of stress and pain associated with wound care affects recovery. Nurs Residential Care. 2010a;12(9):443–6.

Solowiej K, Upton D. The assessment and management of pain and stress in wound care. Br J Community Nurs. 2010b;15(6):S26–33.

Solowiej K, Mason V, Upton D. Psychological stress and pain in wound care, part 3: management. J Wound Care. 2010;19(4):153–5.

Solowiej K, Mason V, Upton D. Review of the relationship between stress and wound healing: part 1. J Wound Care. 2009;18(9):357–66.

Solowiej K, Mason V, Upton D. Psychological stress and pain in wound care, part 3: management. J Wound Care. 2010a;19(4):153–5.

Solowiej K, Mason V, Upton D. Psychological stress and pain in wound care, part 2: a review of pain and stress assessment tools. J Wound Care. 2010b;19(3):110–5.

Soon K, Acton C. Pain-induced stress: a barrier to wound healing. Wounds UK. 2006;2(4):92–101.

Upton D, Solowiej K. Using electronic voting systems in wound care conferences. Wounds UK. 2011;7(1):58–61.

Upton D, South F. The psychological consequences of wounds – a vicious circle that should not be overlooked. Wounds UK. 2011;7(4):136–8.

Upton D, Hender C. The cost of mood disorders in patients with chronic wounds. Wounds UK. 2012;8(1):107–9.

Upton D, Hender C, Solowiej K. Mood disorders in patients with acute and chronic wounds: a health professional perspective. J Wound Care. 2012a;21(1):42–8.

Upton D, Hender C, Solowiej K, Woo K. Stress and pain associated with dressing change in chronic wound patients. J Wound Care. 2012b;22(2):53–61.

Upton D, Solowiej K, Hender C, Woodyat KY. Stress and pain associated with dressing change in patients with chronic wounds. J Wound Care. 2012c;21(2):53–61.

Upton D, Morgan J, Andrews A, et al. The pain and stress of wound treatment in patients with burns. An international burn specialist perspective. Wounds. 2013a;25(8):199–204.

Upton D, Stephens D, Andrews A. Patients' experience of negative pressure wound therapy. J Wound Care. 2013b;22(1):34–9.

Upton D, Thirlaway K. Promoting healthy lifestyles. 2nd ed. London: Routledge; 2014.

Vedhara K, Miles JNV, Wetherell MA, Dawe K, Searle A, Tallon D, Campbell R. Coping style and depression influence the healing of diabetic foot ulcers: observational and mechanistic evidence. Diabetologia. 2010;53(8):1590–8.

Walburn J, Vedhara K, Hankins M, Rixon L, Weinman J. Psychological stress and wound healing in humans: a systematic review and meta-analysis. J Psychosom Res. 2009;67:253–71.

Walshe C. Living with a venous leg ulcer: a descriptive study of patients' experiences. J Adv Nurs. 1995;22(6):1092–100.

Weinman J, Ebrecht M, Scott S, Walburn J, Dyson M. Enhanced wound healing after emotional disclosure intervention. Br J Health Psychol. 2008;13:95–102.

Wilson RH, Wisely JA, Wearden AJ, Dunn KW, Edwards J, Tarrier N. Do illness perceptions and mood predict healing time for burn wounds? A prospective, preliminary study. J Psychosom Res. 2011;71(5):364–6. Epub 2011 Jul 12.

Woo KY. Wound-related pain: anxiety, stress and wound healing. Wounds UK. 2010;6(4):92–8.

Woo KY, Sibbald RG. Chronic wound pain: a conceptual model. Adv Skin Wound Care. 2008;21(4):175–88.

References

Adams C, et al. Isolation by HPLC and characterisation of the bioactive fraction of New Zealand manuka (Leptospermum scoparium) honey. Carbohydr Res. 2008;343(4):651–9.

Anderson JL, Dodman S, Kopelman M, Fleming A. Patient information recall in a rheumatology clinic. Rheumatology. 1979;18(1):18–22.

Bosch JA, Phillips AC, Lord JM, editors. Immunosenescence. NewYork: Springer. 2013. p. 35–46.

Bradlyn AS, Varni JW, Hinds PS. Assessing health-related quality of life in end-of-life care for children and adolescents. In: Field MJ, Behrman RE, editors. When children die: improving palliative and end-of-life care for children and their families. Washington, DC: The National Academies Press; 2003.

Briggs M, Flemming K. Living with leg ulceration: a synthesis of qualitative research. J Adv Nurs. 2007;59(4):319–28.

Christensen AJ, Ehlers SL, Wiebe JS, Moran PJ, Raichle K, Ferneyhough K, et al. Patient personality and mortality: a 4-year prospective examination of chronic renal insufficiency. Health Psychol. 2002;21(4):315–20.

Cohen S, Frank E, Doyle WJ, Skoner DP, Rabin BS, Gwaltney Jr JM. Types of stressors that increase susceptibility to the common cold in adults. Health Psychol. 1998;17:214–23.

Cooper RA, et al. The efficacy of honey in inhibiting strains of Pseudomonas aeruginosa from infected burns. J Burn Care Rehabil. 2002;23:366–70.

Coutts P, Woo K, Bourque S. Treating patients with painful chronic wounds. Nurs Stand. 2008;23(10):42–6.

Dyster-Aas J, Kildal M, Willebrand M. Return to work and health-related quality of life after burn injury. J Rehabil Med. 2007;39(1):49–55.

Eberhardt RT, Raffetto JD. Chronic versus insufficiency. Circulation. 2005;111:2398–409.

Ebrecht M, Hextall J, Kirtley LG, et al. Perceived stress and cortisol levels predict speed of wound healing in healthy male adults. Psychoneuroendocrinology. 2012;29:798–809.

Faurbach JA, Lezotte D, Hills RA, et al. Burden of burn: a norm-based inquiry into the influence of burn size and distress on recovery of physical and psychosocial function. J Burn Care Rehabil. 2005;26(1):8–14.

Favagehi M. Mucosal wound healing is impaired by examination stress. Psychosom Med. 1998;60(3):362–5.

Franks PJ, Moffatt CJ, Doherty DC, et al. Longer-term changes in quality of life in chronic leg ulceration. Wound Repair Regen. 2006;14(5):536–41.

Goodridge D, Trepman E, Embil M. Health-related quality of life in diabetic patients with foot ulcers: Literature review. J Wound Ostomy Continence Nurs. 2005;32(6):368–77.

Gordillo GM, Sen CK. Revisiting the essential role of oxygen in wound healing. Am J Surg. 2003;186(3):259–63.

Greenberg PE, Sisitsky T, Kessler RC, et al. The economic burden of anxiety disorders in the 1990's. J Clin Psychiatry. 1999;60(7):427–35.

Grey JE, Enoch S, Harding KG. ABC of wound healing: wound assessment. BMJ. 2006;332(7536):285.

Heaton PB. Negotiation as an integral part of the physician's clinical reasoning. J Fam Pract. 1981;13:845–8.

Helgeson VS. Social support and quality of life. Qual Life Res. 2003;12(1):25–31.

Higginson IJ, Carr AJ. Using quality of life measures in the clinical setting. BMJ. 2001;1294:322–30.

Leegaard M, Rusteon T, Fagermoen MS. Interference of postoperative pain on women's daily life after early discharge form cardiac surgery. Pain Manag Nurs. 2010;11(2):99–102.

Ley P. Memory for medical information. Br J Soc Clin Psychol. 1979;18:245–55.

Lindsay E, Renyi R, Bawden R. Assessment of wellbeing within the Leg Club network. Poster abstract, Tissue Viability Society, York: UK; 2013.

Lindsay E, Vowden P, Vowden K. Does the anatomical position of the motorcyclist impact venous return? Wounds UK. 2013b; 9(3):46–50.

Lindsay E, Vowden P, Vowden K, Megson J. Motorcycle ride position, venous return and symptoms of chronic venous insufficiency. EWMA J. 2013c;13(1):35–6.

Londahl M, Katzman P, Nilsson A, Christer H. Response to comment on: Londahl et al. Hyperbaric oxygen therapy facilitates healing of chronic foot ulcers in patients with diabetes. Diabetes Care. 2011;33:998–1003.

London School of Economics. The depression report. 2006. Available at: http://cep.lse.ac.uk/textonly/research/mental-health/DEPRESSION_REPORT_LAYARD.pdf.

Mendelson FA, Divino C, Reis ED, Kerstein MD. Wound care after radiation therapy. Adv Skin Wound Care. 2002;15(5):216–24.

Moffatt S, White M, Mackintosh J, Howel D. Using quantitative and qualitative data in health services research: what happens when mixed method findings conflict. BMC Health Serv Res. 2006;6:28.

NICE. Depression in Adults (update). Depression: the treatment and management of depression in adults. Oxford: National Collaborating Centre for Mental Health Commissioned by the National Institute for Health and Clinical Excellence; 2009. p. 13–23.

Richardson C, Upton D. Managing pain and stress in wound care. In: Upton D, editor. Psychological impact of pain in patients with wounds. London: Wounds UK; 2011.

Rippon M, Davies P, Bosanquet N, White RJ. The economic impact of difficult-to-heal venous Leg ulcers and cost effectiveness of treatment options: a review of the published literature. Wounds UK. 2007;3(2):58–73.

Roter D, Hall J. Physician interviewing style and medical information obtained from patients. J Gen Intern Med. 1987;2:326.

Russell D, Cutrona CE, Rose J, Yurko K. Social and emotional loneliness: an examination of Weiss's typology of loneliness. J Pers Soc Psychol. 1984;46(6):1313.

Sarason BR, Shearin EN, Pierce GR, Sarason IG. Interrelations of social support measures: theoretical and practical implications. J Pers Soc Psychol. 1987;52:813–32.

Scheier MF, Matthews KA, Owens JF, Schulz R, Bridges MW, Magovern GJ, et al. Optimism and rehospitalization after coronary artery bypass graft surgery. Arch Intern Med. 1999a;159:829–35.

Scheier MF, Matthews KA, Owens JF, Schulz R, Bridges MW, Magovern GJ, et al. Optimism and rehospitalization after coronary artery bypass graft surgery. Arch Intern Med. 1999b;159:829–35.

Stephen-Haynes J, Gibson B. An evaluation of a two-piece compression hosiery kit within primary care. Poster presentation, Wounds UK Conference, Harrogate; 2006.

Steptoe A, Wardle J, Pollard TM, et al. Stress, social support and health-related behavior: a study of smoking, alcohol consumption and physical exercise. J Psychosom Res. 1996;41:171–80.

Stewart M, Brown JB, Weston WW. Patient-centred medicine. Thousand Oaks: Sage; 1995.

Thomas CM, Morris S. Cost of depression among adults in England in 2000. Br J Psychiatry. 2003;183:514–9.

Upton D, Andrews A, Upton P. Venous leg ulcers: what about wellbeing? J Wound Care. 2014;23(1):14–7.

Van Hecke A, Grypdonck M, Defloor T. Interventions to enhance patient compliance with leg ulcer treatment: a review of the literature. J Clin Nurs. 2008;17(1):29–39.

Van Loey NE, Bremer M, Faber AW, et al. Itching following burns: epidemiology and predictors. Br J Dermatol. 2008;158(1):95–100.

Wahl C, Gregoire JP, Teo K, Beaulieu M, Labelle S, Leduc B, et al. Concordance, compliance and adherence in healthcare: closing gaps and improving outcomes. Healthcare Quaterly. 2005;8(1):65–70.

Wales S. A world of pain. Nurs Stand. 2006;20(36):24–5.

White CE, Renz EM. Advances in surgical care: management of severe burn injury. Crit Care Med. 2008;36(7):S318–24.

WHO. Adherence to long-term therapies: evidence for action. 2003. Available from: http://www.who.int/chp/knowledge/publications/adherence_report/en/.

Williams AM. Issues affecting concordance with leg ulcer care and quality of life. Nurs Stand. 2010;24(45):51–8.

Wolcott RD, Kennedy JP, Dowd SE. Regular debridement is the main tool for maintaining a healthy wound bed in most chronic wounds. J Wound Care. 2009a;18(2):54–6.

Wolcott RD, Gontcharova V, Sun Y, Dowd SE. Evaluation of the bacterial diversity among and within individual venous leg ulcers using bacterial tag-encoded FLX and titanium amplicon pyrosequencing and metagenomic approaches. BMC Microbiol. 2009b;9:226.

Wolf MH, Stiles WB. Further development of the medical interview satisfaction scale. Paper presented at the American Psychological Association Convention, Los Angeles; 1981.

Index

A
Adherence, 171–173

B
Buffer hypothesis, 197
Burn injury
    depression and anxiety, 117
    incidence, 116–117
    model of care, 117–118
    psychological assessment, 120–123
    PTSD, 119
    risk factors, 116
    self-mastery, 119

C
Cardiff wound impact schedule (CWIS), 98, 100
Charing cross venous leg ulcer questionnaire (CCVLUQ), 95
Chronic pain, 28
Cognitive-behavioural therapy (CBT), 49
Communication, 230–231
Compliance, 170–173
Compression bandages
    with footwear, 153
    issues of, 154
    multicomponent, 152–153
    with nurse, 151–152
    surrounding itching and, 154
    for VLU, 149–150
Concordance, 230–231
    adherence, 171–173
    compliance, 170–173
    health belief model, 176–177
    illness perceptions, 178–179
    models of
        cartoon instructions, 175
        communication factors, 175
        Ley's cognitive hypothesis model, 173–174
    patient centred care, 182–183
    patient satisfaction, 181–182
    practice implications, 184–185
    self-care, 177–178
    social support, 179–181

D
Diabetic foot ulcer (DFU)
    amputation risk, 123
    anxiety, 125
    behavioural changes, 127
    conceptual model, 126, 127

Diabetic foot ulcer (*cont.*)
　coping, 125–126
　individuals with, 124
　psychological morbidity, 125
　risk factors, 127–128
Dressing change
　adherence, 145–146
　atraumatic, 146, 147
　conventional, 147, 148
　cotton gauze
　　and bandages, 146
　impact of, 148–149

E
European Wound Management Association (EWMA), 31

F
Faces pain scale, 43–44
Family relationship index (FRI), 198
Family support, 231–232
　caregiver burden, 208
　informal carer, 205
　partner/spouse, 205–207
　unpaid carers, 208

G
Gate control theory (GTC), 33–34
General adaption syndrome (GAS) model
　alarm stage, 60
　exhaustion stage, 61
　physiological, psychological and social factors, 62–63
　resistance stage, 60
General Health Questionnaire (GHQ), 70

H
Health belief model (HBM), 176–177
Health-related quality of life (HRQoL), 225
　assessments, 94
　generic and wound specific measures, 98
　quantitative fixed-response measures, 93
　questionnaires measure, 93–94
　wellbeing, 100
Hospital Anxiety and Depression Scale (HADS), 75
　anxiety and depression, 70–71
　assessment, 71
　physiological measures, 71–73

I
International Association for the Study of Pain (IASP), 27

L
Ley's cognitive hypothesis model, 173–174
Lindsay leg club® model, 202–204

M
McGill pain questionnaire (MPQ), 43

N
Negative pressure wound therapy (NPWT)
　advantages, 155
　clinician reports, 159
　disadvantages, 155

low-pressure, 156
patients' experiences and perceptions, 159–160
quality of life, 156–157
Non-steroidal anti-inflammatory drugs (NSAIDs), 47
Numerical pain rating scale (NPRS), 40

P
Pain, 223–224
assessments, 32, 38
chronic, 28
clinicians and health professionals, 31
cycle of, 35
definition, 27–28
faces pain scale, 43–44
GTC, 33–34
harmful intensity, 28
influencing factors, 36–37
management
analgesic medications, 46–47
assessment, 45–46
multi-modal approach, 46–50
normalisation, 50–51
potential mechanisms of, 49–50
preparation, 44–45
strategies, 48
WHO ladder, 46–47
measurement, 40–42
MPQ, 43
nociceptors, 28–29
non-verbal checklist, 39–40
pathophysiological causes, 38
peripheral neuropathic, 29
phantom, 29, 33
physiological aspects, 36
psychological influences, 38
psychosocial consequences, 3
vs. stress and wound healing
biopsy wounds, 74
chronic levels impact, 76
cortisol assessments, 74
depression and anxiety, 75
impact, 76
importance, 75
indication, 74
negative consequences, 77
photographs and foaming response, 73–74
wound–care professionals, 75
type, 29–30
VAS, 43
VPRS/NPRS, 40
WUWHS, 31–32
Perceived Stress Scale (PSS), 69–70
Peripheral neuropathic pain, 29
Post-traumatic stress disorder (PTSD), 119
Pressure ulcers (PU)
category, 134
classification, 132, 133
domains, 134
impact, 134
phenomenological study, 133
prevention and management, 132
Progressive Muscle Relaxation (PMR), 79
Psychosocial consequences
complex nature, 2–3
daily living limitations, 4–5
disrupted body image, 6–7
emotional and cognitive factors, 13
emotional response, 7–8
exudate and malodour experiences, 3

Psychosocial consequences (*cont.*)
  healing
    implications, 9–13
    process, 3, 6
  health behaviours changes, 8–9
  pain (*see* Pain)
  personal process, 13
  practice implications
    advantages, 17
    chronic wound, 16
    honest information, 16–17
    modern wound care practices, 15
    relaxation technique, 17
  quality of life (*see* Quality of life (QoL))
  resilience, 13–15
  self sense, 6–7
  social
    implications, 3
    isolation, 5–6
  stress (*see* Stress)
  of wounds, 3–4
Psychosocial issues, 221–222

Q
Quality of life (QoL), 225–227
  clinical practice implications
    assessment, 104
    importance, 103–104
  definition, 88
  gap theory, 91–92
  health status and functioning, 89
  HRQoL, 89, 90
  impact factors
    pain (*see* Pain)
    physical functioning, 101–102
    psychological functioning, 102
    social functioning, 102–103
  measurement
    CWIS, 98
    domains, 95–97
    generic and disease specific, 94–95
    patient self-report, 93
    quantitative fixed-response, 93
    questionnaires, 93–94
  NPWT
    Cardiff wound impact schedule, 157
    SF-36 questionnaire, 158
  RCT, 86–87
  social comparison theory, 92
  treatments, 87
  ubiquitous nature, 87

R
Randomised control trials (RCT), 87

S
Social comparison theory, 197–198
Social implications, 3
Social Provisions Scale (SPA), 196
Social support, 231–232
  buffer hypothesis, 197
  concordance, 179–181
  definition, 193–194
  family considerations
    caregiver burden, 208
    informal carer, 205
    partner/spouse, 205–207
    unpaid carers, 208–209
  and health, 198–199
  health impacts, 199–202
  main effect hypothesis, 197
  medical outcomes study-social support survey, 195–196
  social comparison theory, 197–198
  social provisions scale, 196
  sources of, 194–195
  SSQ-SF, 195

Social support questionnaire
(SSQ), 195
State trait anxiety inventory
(STAI), 70
Stress, 224–225
  assessing
    behavioural sign, 66
    GHQ, 70
    HADS, 70–73
    PSS, 69–70
    psychological measures,
      66–68
    STAI, 70
    stress-thermometer,
      66, 69
  GAS model
    alarm stage, 60
    exhaustion stage, 61
    physiological,
      psychological and
      social factors, 62–63
    resistance stage, 60
  healing, 58
  health care, 79–80
  interactional model
    clinical practice, 65
    coping, 65
    description, 64–65
    types, 63
  management, 77–78
  managing stressors, 78–80
  vs. pain and wound healing
    biopsy wounds, 74
    chronic levels impact, 76
    cortisol assessments, 74
    depression and anxiety, 75
    impact, 76
    importance, 75
    indication, 74
    negative consequences, 77
    photographs and foaming
      response, 73–74
    wound–care professionals,
      75
  PMR, 79
  process of, 59
  psychosocial consequences, 3

T
Treatments
  compression bandages
    with footwear, 153
    issues of, 154
    multicomponent, 152–153
    with nurse, 151–152
    surrounding itching and,
      154
    for venous leg ulcer,
      149–150
  dressing change
    adherence, 145–146
    atraumatic dressings, 146,
      147
    conventional dressings,
      147, 148
    cotton gauze and
      bandages, 146
    impact of, 148, 149
  NPWT
    advantages, 155
    clinician reports, 159
    disadvantages, 155
    low-pressure, 156
    patients' experiences and
      perceptions, 160–161
    quality of life, 156–158
    and psychological outcomes,
      228–230

V
Vacuum assisted closure (VAC).
  See Negative pressure
    wound therapy
    (NPWT)
Venous leg ulcers (VLU)
  compression bandages,
    149–150
  impact, 128–129
  nurse–patient relationship, 131
  pain assessment, 131
  physical problems, 128
  qualitative research, 129–130
  reduced mobility, 129–130
  social isolation, 130–131

Verbal pain rating scale (VPRS), 40
Visual analogue scale (VAS), 43

W

Wellbeing, 225–227
  assessment, 104
  clinicians, 106
  CWIS, 100
  definition, 90
  domains, 99
  HRQoL, 100
  hypothesised model, 99–100
  International consensus document (2012), 98–99
  physical and mental health importance, 105
World Health Organisation (WHO), 46–47, 88
World Union of Wound Healing Societies (WUWHS), 31
Wound
  burn injury
    depression and anxiety, 117
    incidence, 116–117
    model of care, 117–118
    psychological assessment, 120–123
    PTSD, 119
    risk factors, 116
    self-mastery, 119
  DFU
    amputation risk, 123
    anxiety, 125
    behavioural changes, 127
    conceptual model, 126, 127
    coping, 125–126
    individuals with, 124
    psychological morbidity, 125
    risk factors, 127–128
  healing *vs.* pain and stress
    biopsy wounds, 74
    chronic levels impact, 76
    cortisol assessments, 74
    depression and anxiety, 75
    impact, 76
    importance, 75
    indication, 74
    negative consequences, 77
    photographs and foaming response, 73–74
    wound–care professionals, 75
  pressure ulcers
    category, 134
    classification, 132, 133
    domains, 134
    impact, 134
    phenomenological study, 133
    prevention and management, 132–133
  VLU
    impact, 128–129
    nurse–patient relationship, 131
    pain assessment, 131
    physical problems, 128
    qualitative research, 129–130
    reduced mobility, 129–130
    social isolation, 130–131

The manufacturer's authorised representative in the EU is Springer Nature Customer Service Centre GmbH, Europaplatz 3, 69115 Heidelberg, Germany. If you have any concerns regarding our products, please contact ProductSafety@springernature.com

Printed and bound by CPI Group (UK) Ltd, Croydon, CR0 4YY
23/03/2026
02076657-0001